# Understanding Child Sexual Abuse

Understanding Health and Sickness Series
*Miriam Bloom, Ph.D.*
*General Editor*

# Understanding Child Sexual Abuse

Edward L. Rowan, M.D.

University Press of Mississippi
Jackson

www.upress.state.ms.us

The University Press of Mississippi is a member of the Association of
American University Presses.

Copyright © 2006 by University Press of Mississippi
All rights reserved
Manufactured in the United States of America

First edition 2006

Illustrations by Alan Estridge

Library of Congress Cataloging-in-Publication Data

Rowan, Edward L.
    Understanding child sexual abuse / Edward L. Rowan.— 1st ed.
        p. cm. — (Understanding health and sickness series)
    Includes bibliographical references and index.
    ISBN 1-57806-806-1 (cloth : alk. paper) — ISBN 1-57806-807-X
(pbk. : alk. paper)
    1. Child sexual abuse. 2. Child sexual abuse—Treatment. I. Title.
II. Series.
    RC560.C56R69    2006
    362.76—dc22                                     2005018087

British Library Cataloging-in-Publication Data available

# Contents

# Introduction

There are two sides to every story. The issue of child sexual abuse is no exception. In this book I will explore the dynamics, effects, and treatment options available to both the children and the adults involved. Broadly speaking, child sexual abuse refers to sex forced on a child by an older person. With a few exceptions, the objective is the sex itself. Power and humiliation are the objectives of rape and the sexual assaults common in prisons and military organizations, and they are not part of this discussion.

The language we use to describe what happens between participants in a sexual experience has a built-in bias. The terms *sexual abuse, sexual molestation,* and *child rape* have a negative connotation, as do *victim* and *survivor. Predator, perpetrator, molester, rapist, child abuser, deviant,* and *pedophile* are also negative terms. Language bias influences the way information is processed and it is difficult to feel positive about any of these terms. Despite this, I will retain those terms because of their pervasive use in the scientific and lay literature.

The people who work with clinical populations of damaged victims and survivors are justifiably angry at those who caused the damage. They also seem to believe that adults who have sex with children are using them as substitutes for the adults they are incompetent to have or to hold. They believe that such people deserve no sympathy and should be despised. For many in the larger Judeo-Christian perspective, the only justification for sexual activity is procreation within the sanctity of marriage. The sentimental image that children are innocents to be cherished provides additional justification for despising the child abuser.

University of Hamburg, Germany, psychologist Gunter Schmidt believes that the negative view about sex with children relates not to the sex itself but to the evolution of what he calls "consensual morality." If two people of equal power knowingly and willingly agree to do something sexual, then it is acceptable. Conservatives do not believe that children can mutually consent and liberals focus on the perceived power imbalance, so that adults who have sex with children have no supporters except each other.

One complicating factor here is that we live in a society where children are sexualized in the media. Advertisements for jeans are only one example of young girls in provocative poses. Does anyone really believe that a beauty contest for four-year-olds where the contestants have teased hair and makeup and sing "I Wanna Make Love to You" is all about college scholarships? Where is the outrage when children are exploited in that way?

Another factor is the growing body of research that indicates that while adult-child sex is legally and morally wrong, it is not inevitably harmful. To assume that it is always problematic helps create "victims" where there may be none and, in the extreme, creates "abusers" where there may be none either.

Clinicians who work with offenders see this world differently. They know that there are many reasons why adults have sex with children. They strive to understand how each individual comes to behave in the ways that he or she does and, if possible, to tailor a treatment program for that person. Their objective is to stop repetitive behavior so that other children will be safe if and when the perpetrator returns to society.

In this volume we look first at the men and women who become abusers. We consider the bases for their sexual arousal by children, their emotional bonds with children, their lack of adult opportunities, and the factors that cause them to lose control over their sexual urges. We look at particular groups such as priests and incest offenders and at organizations that promote sex with children.

Determination of the true incidence and prevalence of child sexual abuse, discussed in chapter 2, is difficult because of the wide variability in sampling techniques. Clinical and legal samples are not representative of the population as a whole. The true incidence of problems that result from the sexual contact is generally overestimated. In some cases, problems can be created by therapeutic interventions themselves.

For some individuals, the effects of sexual victimization are devastating and often manifest as post-traumatic stress disorder. Chapter 3 examines the great deal of work now being done in an effort to understand the neurobiological correlates of this disorder. Childhood abuse can also damage trust, self-confidence, faith, and the capacity for intimacy later on. There is some evidence that maladaptive personality styles may also be the result of early sexual abuse.

The treatment of survivors follows that for post-traumatic stress disorder: recognize the trauma, control the response to it, and integrate it into life experience. Chapter 4 will consider the recovered memory controversy and particular treatments including psychotherapy, sex therapy, cognitive behavioral therapy, and eye movement desensitization and reprocessing.

A number of sophisticated programs for the treatment of sex offenders are discussed in chapter 5. Most of them attempt to change arousal patterns and build skills for better adult relationships and community integration. There is not a great deal of evidence that they actually change the recidivism rate. Those individuals most likely to reoffend before treatment are still likely to reoffend after it.

The prevention of child sexual abuse, an elusive goal, is examined in chapter 6. Most programs address "stranger danger" despite the fact that the vast majority of offenders are known to their victims. Organizations such as the Catholic Church and Boy Scouts of America have developed preventive measures to protect both the children and the adults in their programs. Sex offender registries are now required in every state; their value, however, is limited.

Chapter 7 discusses groundbreaking work in the neurobiology of trauma responses that may help to determine which factors are associated with increased vulnerability or increased resilience to traumatic events. Some of this work applies to offenders as well. Brain imaging to determine which areas are activated or deactivated and genetic studies of various neurotransmitters are part of this research.

In thirty years of work with both victims and offenders, I have seen both sides of the story. I hope that this volume will enable the reader to develop a real understanding of the multiple meanings of child sexual abuse.

# Understanding Child Sexual Abuse

# 1. Who Becomes an Abuser?

Each of us is the product of a lifelong series of sexual turn-ons and turn-offs, some reinforced and practiced, some banished from conscious thought, and some resisted every day. Sigmund Freud used the expression *polymorphous perverse* to describe the primitive sexual urges in all of us. Our natural and normal sexual urges become associated with what is happening in the world around us and, in terms of simple behavioral conditioning, events become paired with those sexual urges and become interpreted as sexual turn-ons. Given the right circumstances, any man or woman might become aroused by men, women, children, multiple partners, or animals. Humiliation, power, bondage, or special or specific objects or items of clothing may also become a source of arousal. Potentially then, we might all have "deviant" arousal patterns; most of us, however, choose not to act on them.

Sexual arousal becomes a problem when it leads to the involvement of an unwilling participant. Looking at a centerfold is different from peeking through a window at an unwilling neighbor. Being aroused by underwear is different from stealing that underwear from an unattended laundry basket. A couple may choose to tie one or the other partner to the bed as part of their lovemaking, but that is different from binding an unwilling victim.

Sexual assault is very broadly defined as unwanted sexual contact with another person. Sexual assault on a child, or child molestation, is more narrowly defined but the definition varies from one legal jurisdiction to another. The bottom line is that a child cannot knowingly or willingly consent to a sexual relationship with a more powerful, older person. Depending on the jurisdiction, to be charged with molestation, the older person must be at least sixteen or eighteen and at least three or five years older than the child. This acknowledges that sexual experimentation between younger peers does exist but that sexual contact between a child and an adult man or woman is wrong. However, violation of a social norm does not inevitably equate with harm to the child.

Not all child sexual abusers are pedophiles. The Diagnostic and Statistical Manual of the American Psychiatric Association, 4th Edition (DSM IV), defines *pedophilia* as one of the *paraphilias* or recurrent and intense sexual urges and sexually arousing fantasies under "deviant" circumstances. Here, *deviant* refers to nonhuman objects of desire, suffering or humiliation by the person or partner, or involvement of children or other non-consenting persons. Pedophiles are aroused by and fantasize almost exclusively about prepubescent children. *Ephebophile* is a term used to describe people who are aroused by pubescent or early adolescent children. Individuals who have sex with children without the exclusive urge and/or fantasy would not technically, then, be pedophiles or ephebophiles. A true pedophile or ephebophile, on the other hand, might have urges and fantasies about sex with children and never act on them. Two alleged examples of this are the respected nineteenth-century British academicians Charles Dodgson (Lewis Carroll) and Sir James Barrie. Both apparently fantasized exclusively about children but sublimated those urges into writing about Alice in Wonderland and Peter Pan, respectively.

Seen from this perspective, "child sexual abuse" is a social construct. Our society believes that sexual contact between adults and children is wrong. It does not matter that the ancient Greeks waxed poetic about men having sex with boys or that in some cultures children were introduced to sexual behavior by designated relatives. It does not matter that child prostitutes approach men in the streets. It does not matter that children are naturally curious about sexuality. It does not matter that the abuser can rationalize or blame the victim, saying, for example, that the child asked for it, it was educational, or the devil made him do it. No such rationale is valid in this social context. What does matter is that sex with children is an abuse of power. There are, however, a number of studies of boys who initiated sex with adults and felt that they possessed the power in the relationship. Despite this perception, the adult would have been criminally liable if discovered.

Historically there have been a number of attempts to classify and understand the people who have sex with children. Nicholas Groth, a psychologist with the Connecticut Department of Corrections, differentiated between so-called fixated and regressed pedophiles. According to his theory, some people never mature and the objects of their sexual desire remain the same as when they were children themselves. They never grow to develop a sexual interest in adults and their arousal is arrested or fixated on young children. Others have "normal" adult sexual relationships but various stressors might cause them to return or regress to an earlier immature sexual interest in children. By our definition, this group might not even be considered true pedophiles. Both patterns occur and the difference is important because there is hope for controlling future bad behavior in the latter group. Another theory holds that there is a special dynamic in incestuous families and that this form of sexual behavior is different from sexual assault by strangers. One erroneous belief is that an interest in children is part of a homosexual orientation. Some people believe that there might be a genetic predisposition or other physical explanation for attraction to children. No single formulation is helpful in understanding why some adults have sex with some children. Both men and women may be abusers and they may be so for different reasons.

In the 1980s Sharon Araji and David Finkelhor at the University of New Hampshire developed a comprehensive model to explain the dynamics of child sexual abuse. After reviewing many studies, they determined that significant variables in the behavior pattern formed four clusters: sexual arousal, emotional congruence, blockage, and disinhibition. Their elegant system has not been widely adopted because many child advocates mistakenly believe that it shifts the blame to the victim. This is only one example of how clinicians who come to the area of child sexual abuse as child advocates see the world differently from those who try to understand the perpetrator.

The Araji-Finkelhor model postulates that elements from each of the four clusters must be present for sexual abuse of children to occur.

*Sexual arousal.* Not everyone finds children sexually attractive or even believes that children can be sexual objects. Those who do have often had sexual experiences when they were children themselves and have grown up in a family or culture that condoned the view of children as sexual objects. This so-called cycle of abuse is not inevitable and is actually less common than might be assumed. The majority of child victims do not become abusers, but some do. Sexual behavior itself is not necessarily arousing. An object or behavior becomes arousing when it is associated with the positive experience of pleasure. The most common pleasure in this context is orgasm, and the most common way to achieve orgasm is through masturbation. Masturbation is a completely normal activity known to almost everyone. Few of us masturbate with an empty mind, and the fantasies that routinely and reliably turn us on have been reinforced, sometimes hundreds of times, by a pleasurable orgasm. For most of us, the fantasy objects mature as we do, but if the recurrent fantasy object is an idealized child rather than an idealized young adult centerfold, then the person who has such a fantasy might be at increased risk for acting on it. Studies that monitor sexual arousal have shown that many adolescents and adults respond positively to pictures of children as well as adults. The potential for sexual arousal to children is greater than we might imagine, but few people collect pornographic images of children and even fewer produce them for sexual gratification.

When the United States Supreme Court was asked in 1964 to define pornography, Justice Potter Stewart famously replied, "I shall not today attempt to define [it] . . . but I know it when I see it." Pornographic material is that which appeals to one's prurient interest, but not everyone's prurient interest is the same. In 1970 the U.S. Commission on Pornography found the material itself to be harmless. Looking at pictures does not cause deviant behavior; those individuals with deviant arousal seek appropriate pictures. The reason that there is a wide range of material available in any commercial sex shop is that pornography is an individual preference associated with individual arousal patterns. A man turned on by garter belts and high heels would probably not be turned on by animal images. A pedophile would have no interest in images of adults having intercourse unless, perhaps, a woman had small breasts and shaved her pubic hair or a man had shaved his body hair. When high-quality commercial pornography is not available, many individuals will produce their own images. This is especially true for pedophiles, as child pornography is illegal. Many normal adults will be sexually aroused by a variety of stimuli, including images of children.

Many deviant adults will respond to a range of stimuli as well, but pedophiles appear to be an exception—their primary interest is children. Child pornography is illegal and does not appeal to everyone; therefore, the possession or collection of such material seems to be a reliable indicator of a persistent and acknowledged arousal pattern. It is important to understand that, for those who do find children sexually arousing, this arousal feels perfectly natural and they wonder how people could be aroused in any other way. They may realize that others do not approve, but this does not make the urge any less compelling. A classic literary example of this is Vladimir Nabokov's Professor Humbert Humbert, whose loving descriptions and driven pursuit of his "nymphet" Lolita serve to act out his fixated preadolescent fantasies about a girl named Annabel.

*Emotional congruence.* Most of us no longer identify emotionally with children or try to relate to them as equals. For some, however, it is more comforting and satisfying to act like a child or to be with children. The most obvious explanations for this are developmental delays and immaturity, but those with chronic low self-esteem and lack of self-confidence are simply more comfortable relating to children than to adults. These are not adults who coach or teach children how to play a game; these are adults who join in the game as peers.

*Blockage.* Some adults who are sexually attracted to children do have a committed relationship with another adult. Most do not, and for many of those who do, sex is not part of that relationship. A man may fail to be turned on because adults are not sexually arousing; he may feel inadequate as an adult partner because of erectile dysfunction or premature or delayed ejaculation. His partner may be sexually unavailable because of physical or emotional absence or disability, sexual dysfunction such as problems with arousal, pain, or orgasm, or a conflict in the relationship. Failure to establish an adult relationship may be the result of choice or the consequence of inadequate social skills to establish and maintain one. In some cases, a person is unable to maintain an intimate bond with another adult. This inability to bond may be due to circumstances where the first interactions with caregivers were characterized by neglect, rejection, physical abuse, or perceived abandonment and the child failed to attach to those important people. When the child felt bad for whatever reason, there was no one available for support. These individuals grow up without positive relationships in their lives and without the capacity to develop close bonds with others. Some abusers maintain a sexually appropriate adult relationship for show and continue to seek sexual gratification from children.

*Disinhibition.* The fourth factor simply means that the desire to have sex with children is not controlled or inhibited. There can be many reasons for this. Cultural or family rules may not prohibit and may even encourage sexual contact between children and adults so that the need to avoid such behavior is not internalized. If bonding with an infant is a powerful inhibitor of future sexual abuse, then fathers who are absent or stepfathers or mothers' boyfriends who have no early relationship with the child are more at risk to abuse that child later in life. Some individuals may take advantage of opportunities for sexual behavior with children because of poor impulse control. A severe mental illness manifest as delusional thinking or memory impairment may override previously well-established boundaries. Drug and/or alcohol intoxication may result in short-term suspension of boundaries, as may acutely stressful situations such as death, divorce, or job loss. Obviously, more than one of these conditions can occur at the same time.

Within the framework of these dynamics, there are many paths to becoming a sexual abuser. One perpetrator who has achieved exceptional notoriety of late has been the "pedophile priest." The John Jay College of Criminal Justice study of all priests in the country was reported to the United States Conference of Catholic Bishops in February 2004. The investigators found that approximately four percent of priests had sexually abused a minor child in the last fifty years. Most of the men had graduated from seminary before 1979. At that time young boys were encouraged to retreat from society to a community of similar young men who were indoctrinated with the idea that sexual activity was the original sin. Their sexual identity became "fixed" at the time they left the outside world. When they finally returned to society, they were sexual twelve-year-olds in the bodies of adult priests. The priestly culture of celibacy made no provision for adult sexual relationships and the objects of their sexual interest were children. When a priest did offend, he was usually reassigned and protected by the hierarchy so that, on average, it was twenty-five years before the abuse was reported.

A. W. Richard Sipe, a psychotherapist and former priest, has worked extensively with abusive priests. He attributes much of the problem of abuse to what he calls the "homosocial" secret world of the priesthood—a sexually immature, all-male culture of power and reward. Often inadequately prepared in the higher meaning of celibacy, young priests are left to struggle alone with their preadolescent and adolescent sexual conflicts. According to Sipe, some later abusive behavior by these priests may be attributed to their own adolescent experimentation, some to the culture of abuse in some seminaries, and some to the inherently "evil" ones who choose the vocation for the powerful role of "Father" and easy access to children. Priests are trusted and so have easy access to children.

Other predatory abusers have to work harder to be close to them. They may supervise youth groups or coach youth sports. But they still have to isolate potential victims. Most discover tricks that work for them and evolve into modi operandi. First, they must identify potential victims and test them for vulnerability.

Children gather around when someone takes a puppy to the park. A "steady ender" who always holds the end of the rope and never wants to jump is always welcome on the playground. Kids feel special when an adult wants to play catch or ride bikes with them. A relationship can develop in an Internet chat room where some adults try to pass as children while others openly solicit sex. Once a child has shown interest, the predator begins to test the limits of invasion of personal space. He does this in such a way that he can deny the true intention. "Sorry, I didn't mean to touch you." If the child does not resist then there are invitations for a ride home, or ice cream, or special time together to isolate the child from others and create an opportunity for the sexual approach. The adult characterizes the child as special but, paradoxically, as someone who would never be believed if a parent were told. The perpetrator often rationalizes his behavior in terms of education for the child or as a response to a child's need for closeness. Molesters often believe that children initiate sexual contact and consent to it.

Youth groups such as Boy Scouts, Boys' Clubs, and Big Brothers are often the targets of pedophiles. The boys are there and access is easy. Parents are not always involved in these programs and it is relatively easy to isolate vulnerable boys—especially in a tent on a campout far from observation. Boys looking for role models instead meet predators. Common approaches to lure boys into intimate relationships include massage, initiation rites, pornography, and alcohol.

For many years, the Boy Scouts in particular played down the problem. Their priority was damage control and the avoidance of bad publicity and the potential loss of members. When they learned of abuse, local Scouters asked the perpetrator to resign but usually failed to report the abuse to the police. For decades, the national office of the Boy Scouts of America maintained a confidential file of men who should not be allowed in the program; however, reports to that file from the field were haphazard and, according to freelance journalist Patrick Boyle, the man in charge of those files never read them anyway. Abusers would simply move to another area and rejoin the program.

In the late 1980s a series of high profile lawsuits allowed the public to see the confidential files. By then this file contained the names of nearly two thousand men who should not be allowed to rejoin. Only then did the Scouts take steps to educate their membership about the potential danger within their ranks.

One group of molesters without an access problem is the one that abuses children within the family. *Intrafamilial sexual abuse* is a better term than incest because authority and trust within a household are more important factors than the biological relationship between the individuals concerned. The dynamics of sexual acting-out within families are as varied as the dynamics of any other form of child sexual abuse. One important factor appears to be the failure to develop the nurturing, protective bond thought to be characteristic of parents. Male abusers are often absent and fail to bond with the child when it is an infant. They also feel incredibly entitled to control their households. Sexual abuse of a child is often part of a pervasive pattern of physical and sexual abuse in the home, often in the context of intoxication. Wives are beaten and sexually abused. Pets are tortured. Children who intervene often meet the same fate, but they might even without intervening. If a mother is absent, a child or series of children may be forced to take on maternal duties, including that of sexual partner. It is striking how often mothers appear to be unaware that a child or succession of children is being abused. Abusers often blame the child as deserving of punishment because they are bad or promiscuous. Pledges to secrecy and threats of retribution for disclosure are nearly universal.

Springfield, Massachusetts, psychologist Denise Gelinas has described an intrafamilial pattern she calls the "parentified child": a child, usually the oldest daughter, functioning in a maternal role. This pattern may carry on for generations. Mother marries a dependent, immature man who needs to be taken care of. When she has children of her own and childcare becomes physically and emotionally exhausting, she withdraws from her husband. He feels angry, abandoned, and incapable of supporting her. As they withdraw from each other, he escalates his demand for nurturance. The situation worsens with each new child in the family.

Mother then turns to the oldest child for support and assistance in meeting the family's needs. She withdraws more from her husband, who now seeks nurturance from the parentified daughter. This is especially true if the father is not confident enough or feels restrained from developing relationships outside the family. The demand may escalate if the father suffers a loss of support or self-esteem such as the death of a parent, loss of a job, personal injury, or birth of yet another child. At first the daughter will try to meet his emotional needs: she asks about his day, listens, and tries to comfort him. If he then shows poor judgment, impulsivity, or an enhanced sense of entitlement, and especially if alcohol is a factor, the relationship may proceed to physical intimacy as well. The father confuses sexual contact with nurturance.

The daughter keeps her secret from the mother because she is responsible for mother's well-being as well as father's. Guilt, low self-esteem, and lost childhood are the consequences. The pattern becomes internalized and she may well choose a husband who is dependent, exploitive, and abusive—just like her father. Her daughter may then fall into the same role and the pattern will continue for generations.

There are common elements in these patterns even though the paths to the sexual abuse of children differ. The abuser first acknowledges children as sexual objects, either in their own right or as substitutes for adults, and then makes an emotional connection with the child to satisfy his own unmet needs. He typically lacks a meaningful adult sexual relationship and fails to develop a social conscience that says that sex with children is wrong, or an intervening variable causes previously good judgment to be temporarily or permanently suspended.

When women molest children, the dynamics are different. The definition of a pedophile as one in whom "the act or fantasy of engaging in sexual activity with prepubescent children as the preferred or exclusive method of achieving sexual excitement" rarely applies. In fact, there are essentially no reports in the literature of women who meet that definition. There are reports of female teachers having sexual relationships with male students, but none of those women have been examined by a mental health professional who then wrote up the case and determined that they were true pedophiles. Several years ago, my colleagues and I looked at the records of nine women who were evaluated for child sexual abuse. The other 591 records in the sample, or 98.5 percent of the accused, were men. The most striking feature was that most of the women offended in the company of a dominant male partner who instigated the abuse. They also tended to display

significant emotional or intellectual impairment that inter-
fered with nurturing and bonding behavior and suspended
their judgment about what was appropriate contact with their
children.

The cycle of abuse is not a universal phenomenon. Every
abused child does not go on to become an abusive adult.
Only one-third of male offenders report having been victims
themselves. A 2001 British study followed abused boys into
adulthood and identified only twelve percent who became
abusers. These individuals often had a history of family violence, maternal neglect, and abuse by a woman as well. Abusing others is most common among adolescent males and
females for whom abuse is either a model of interaction with
younger children or a way to master their own sense of being
out of control. Abusing women rarely report a personal history
of abuse.

Most adults who are sexually attracted to children have
internalized the societal prohibition of such behavior and do
not act on that attraction. Others want to overturn that prohibition. The North American Man-Boy Love Association
(NAMBLA) puts itself forward as an advocacy group for a
misunderstood minority group like gays or transsexuals. Their
website states that their mission is to "end oppression of men
and boys who have mutually consensual relationships."

It is instructive to quote from NAMBLA material: "Boys
often approach sex with great interest and enthusiasm, so that
consensual sexual experiences are not harmful. . . . Once sexual experiences have become known to others, secondary harm
to youngsters can be induced by inappropriate reactions of
parents, police, social workers, lawyers and other adults, where
no apparent harm results from the sexual contact itself. . . . If
people are not taught to despise their bodies and fear sex, if
their sexual choices are not forced upon them by others, and

if they are not subjected to harsh or stigmatizing reactions to their sexual choices and experiences, they will not be harmed by having sex, regardless of how old or young they are or with whom they have sex." The site goes on with glowing testimonials from boys who thought that sex with men was a wonderful, positive experience. At one time, the site recommended that members join the Boy Scouts for easy access to children. There is also a so-called Women's Auxiliary of NAMBLA that supports consensual relationships between women and girls.

Proponents of adult-child sex often point out that such relationships have been perfectly acceptable at some times and in some cultures. Until the late nineteenth century, the age of consent in England was ten. Current Dutch law gives twelve as the age of consent for sex. There have been several societies where adult-child sex was seen not as gratifying adult desires but as beneficial to the child. Early explorers noted that the receipt of adult semen was believed to facilitate growth and development among the Siwans of North Africa, Aranda of Australia, Marquesans, Tahitians, and Etoro and Kaluli of New Guinea. Child brides have been given in ancient China and elsewhere to solidify political and social alliances. The ultimate goal was that the bride produce a child; however, the timing for that was apparently left up to the husband. In Cameroun, sex with a child is seen not as sexual abuse but as a property crime and is punished by having to make a payment to the child's family. When they reach puberty, young girls are frequently given in marriage in polygamous sects in the western United States, some Muslim sects, and some gypsy tribes. Western culture, however, finds adult-child sex unacceptable.

Sex with children is still legal, or at least not actively discouraged, in some parts of the world. Child prostitutes usually come from the poorest class of a society and may be homeless and drug-dependent. Some are sold by their parents or kidnapped, and selling sex becomes an economic necessity for them. A prostitute in Thailand makes twenty-five times as much as she would in most other occupations.

An estimated half million prostitutes in Thailand are under age 16, 40 percent younger than eleven. There are nearly as many in India, where an even higher percentage is younger. With around sixty thousand child prostitutes, the Philippines is a distant third in Southeast Asia. Most of these prostitutes are girls, but in Sri Lanka an estimated thirty thousand boys are in the trade. Brazil leads South America in child prostitution with perhaps as many as half a million children, both boys and girls, selling sex. The practice also appears to be growing in Colombia and Benin.

Because child prostitution may be culturally acceptable in these areas (e.g., 75 percent of Thai males have paid for sex with a prostitute) it has become the attraction for what has come to be known as "sex tourism." At one time, joining a tour group to Bangkok to have sex with kids was no more difficult than going to Orlando to see Mickey and Goofy. For those patrons the desire for a virginal, disease-free child partner was as much a fantasy as Peter Pan. United States government outrage over the practice has caused some of these countries to be less hospitable to sex-seeking tourists, but for economic reasons the practice is not likely to go away.

It is probably not necessary for a pedophile to travel to South America or Southeast Asia for sex with a child. A 2003 Norwegian survey of all the adolescents in school in Oslo reported that 1.4 percent had sold sex. More boys than girls were sellers and more than half had done so more than ten times. The researchers suggested that the rate among adolescents who were no longer in school might be much higher, as the sellers still in school also acknowledged problems with delinquent behavior and the use of alcohol and drugs. These problems are more frequent in dropouts. It is quite likely that every city in the United States has a group of such children—homeless, drug-dependent, and selling sex in order to survive.

Proponents of adult-child sex often argue that children desire sexual self-determination. While it is true that children have always experimented and rehearsed sexual behaviors with peers, this is not the same as exploitation by adults. Children neither develop the same sexual scripts nor recognize the same sexual meanings as adults. To them, a kiss is just a kiss.

# 2. Who Is at Risk?

In child sexual abuse, the more powerful adult takes advantage of the weakness he sees in the child. Being an altar server for an abusive priest, attending a day care center run by an abusive operator, playing for a pedophile Little League coach, or hugging a too-friendly uncle are all activities that put children at a higher risk of abuse; however, not all children in such circumstances become victims. A strong sense of right and wrong, self-confidence, and a willingness to resist and then to report inappropriate behavior all protect against abuse. These same characteristics may also lessen the traumatic response if abuse does occur. Children who lack these attributes are at risk.

No child asks to be sexually abused. Many are. Determining the exact incidence of child sexual abuse is difficult, but surveys have generally found that 10 to 15 percent of American men and 15 to 25 percent of American women were exposed to at least one unwanted sexual experience as children. There appears to be no difference in incidence based on ethnic background. Rates of abuse among African Americans, Hispanic Americans, and Native Americans are the same as those for non-Hispanic white Americans, although individuals, families, and cultural groups may process the experience differently. These differences would be a fruitful area for research.

In 1974 the Child Abuse Prevention and Treatment Act made reporting mandatory in all states. The requirement to report suspected abuse applies to health-care workers, school personnel, childcare providers, social workers, law enforcement officers, and mental health professionals; some states include film processors, emergency medical technicians, and firefighters.

Eighteen states require any person who suspects abuse to report it. Reporting overrides all privileged and confidential communications except those between attorney and client. Clergy privilege (formerly known as priest-penitent privilege) takes many confusing forms. Most states exempt information obtained in confession from mandatory reporting, but they may or may not except "spiritual advice" or the even more vague "communication made in a professional capacity." Fifteen states (Alabama, Alaska, Arkansas, Georgia, Hawaii, Iowa, Kansas, New York, Ohio, South Carolina, South Dakota, Vermont, Virginia, Washington, and Wisconsin) had no obligation for clergy to report abuse in 2003.

"Were you sexually abused as a child?" A survey question like this one elicits a variety of responses, depending upon a number of factors including exactly how the question is phrased, who asks it, and who answers it. The range of activities included in "child sexual abuse" is the first variable. Sometimes the surveyor provides a specific list of sexual activities, but respondents often must decide the definition for themselves. Normal sexual experimentation before age twelve and consensual sexual activity between peers should be excluded. One survey's "sexual experience" might include seductive speech, verbal solicitation, sexual talk, or exposure to a "flasher." Another's "sexual contact" might include kissing or fondling. Fondling may or may not include non-genital touch. Some people do not consider oral or anal contact as real sex. Others do not consider that sex has occurred without penetration. The wide variety of definitions does not minimize the potential impact of any of these behaviors on the victim, as all may have lasting consequences; however, variable definitions make it difficult to compare studies and to determine the true incidence of abusive behavior.

Information gathered in a face-to-face interview where there is clarification and followup in the context of a dialogue differs from that gathered on an anonymous questionnaire. Individuals may give a negative response to a general question but provide a more positive response when asked a specific question. Male and female interviewers are given different responses to the same question. The life experiences of undergraduate students in introductory psychology courses are different from those of the general public. Surveys of patients in a community mental-health center or hospital emergency room provide more positive responses to questions about sexual abuse. Patients in a sexual-dysfunction clinic acknowledge the highest rates of abuse of all.

Remote events are more difficult to recall than recent ones. A complicating factor is the demonstrated inconsistency in adolescent reporting of any sexual behavior. In one study of 217 adolescents in a STD (sexually transmitted disease) clinic, eighty-one reported a history of sexual abuse on their initial interview but only fifty-four answered the same questions positively seven months later. Stress at the time of response and a changing relationship to the questioner are possible explanations for the variable responses, but the responses vary nonetheless.

Younger children who report sexual abuse may be even more inconsistent in their narratives. They may be more suggestible when interviewed by poorly trained investigators. They may also be more easily caught up in the mass hysteria of accusations of alleged preschool or day-care sexual abuse. The use of anatomically correct dolls was once considered an essential part of such interviews; however, playing with such dolls is not part of the average child's experience and curiosity about the dolls may contaminate the fact-finding interview.

They are no longer in common use. Hysterical reports of escalating sexual abuse culminating in satanic rituals and murder should be particularly suspect. The FBI has never documented a case of ritualistic satanic child sexual abuse and murder in the United States. Accusations that arise as part of custody disputes must be taken seriously, but also considered in context. Shortcomings in survey and interview methodology must not detract from the fact that millions of children in the U.S. experience sexual contact with adults each year.

One of the better recent statistical studies was done by sociologist Edward Laumann and his colleagues at the University of Chicago in the early 1990s. They studied a representative sample of the general population of the United States and found that 12 percent of males and 17 percent of females had been "sexually touched when children." They specifically excluded non-touching behaviors such as exhibitionism and restricted the definition of "contacts" to those by persons older than fourteen with persons younger than twelve. All age groups reported the same percentage of sexual touch, suggesting that there has been no change in the actual rate of child sexual abuse over the years. Girls were most often touched by men and more often by adult men than by adolescents. Their most vulnerable age range was seven to ten. Boys were more likely to be touched by adolescent females, followed in frequency by adolescent males and then by adult males. Boys tended to be older than girls when victimized and were more likely to have had vaginal intercourse with female abusers than girls were with male abusers. Approximately 70 percent of both men and women reported that they were victims of a single abuser, even though there may have been many instances of abuse. Victims knew the vast majority of abusers as family friends or relatives; only 4 to 7 percent of child sexual abusers were strangers.

By contrast, a similar study done in Britain at the same time was seriously flawed. The surveyors did not ask about masturbation because it was "embarrassing." They did not ask about childhood sexual experience and eliminated any data about "first intercourse" prior to age thirteen because it was "inappropriate to the task." The resulting compilation of sexual behavior in Britain was not useful for comparison.

Gelinas noted that intrafamilial abuse is usually initiated when the child is between the ages of four and nine. Younger children are more compliant and may believe that what is happening to them is really just affection or training. They are also more susceptible to threats and bribes. Abusers exploit the child's loyalty, need for affection, desire to please, and trust. Before the age of eleven or twelve the sexual behavior is usually limited to fondling or oral-genital contact. Vaginal insertion is difficult with a prepubescent girl. Anal insertion does happen.

The abusive behavior in Gelinas's sample was limited to a single incident in 17 percent of cases, lasted less than six months in 24 percent, six to twelve months in 19 percent, one to five years in 31 percent, and more than five years in 9 percent. Gelinas noted that the abuse usually ended at age fourteen or fifteen when the victim realized that such behavior was wrong and was able to spend more time away from home. More force would have been required to continue the abuse and the perpetrators were not prepared to apply it.

Child sexual abuse may result in psychopathology in some individuals, but it does not follow that every incident of abuse produces a psychological disorder. Many studies have been done to survey healthy populations and determine how many people in the sample had sexual experiences as children and how many developed psychological problems. In July 1998 Bruce Rind at Temple University and colleagues wrote an article entitled "A meta-analytic examination of assumed properties of child sexual abuse among college samples" in the *Psychological Bulletin*, a publication of the American Psychological Association (APA). A meta-analysis is not new research but a method of employing common statistics to compare and compile data from previously published studies. These psychologists tried to test the premise that in a population with a history of child sexual abuse, this exposure would cause intense psychological harm on a widespread basis for both sexes. They examined fifty-nine studies with a combined sample size of nearly sixteen thousand college students, both male and female. Fourteen percent of the men and 27 percent of the women reported a history of child sexual abuse. They looked for correlations of the incidence of child sexual abuse with eighteen symptom clusters, including eating disorders, depression, anxiety, dissociation, sexual adjustment, and somatization, and found that the frequency of problems in the abused group was not different from that in the group that had not been abused. They factored in severity of abuse, factored out adverse family situations such as family violence, conflict, and lack of support, and still found no correlation. When the sexual contact had been experienced as consensual, a significant percentage of respondents (11 percent of the women and 37 percent of the men) thought the experience was positive. Similar percentages reported their response as neutral. Women forced into an incestuous relationship did have more distress, but this was often temporary. The group concluded that while child sexual abuse was morally and legally wrong and obviously devastating to some individuals, it was not inherently and inevitably harmful. They then went on to make what would be a very controversial suggestion: Do not label every single incident as abuse; call it by the value-neutral term "adult-child sex" unless it results in problems. These findings were consistent with research that found that the vast majority of adults exposed to trauma do not develop post-traumatic stress disorder.

The report that every incident of "abuse" did not cause irreparable harm was met with skepticism by some people, including individuals who accused Rind and the APA of praising pedophilia. The situation was further exacerbated when NAMBLA praised the article on its website. Under intense pressure including the first-ever Congressional resolution condemning a scientific study, the APA apologized for publishing the paper. Irate member psychologists then accused the APA of abandoning good social science in favor of political appeasement. Ultimately, the APA retracted the retraction, but the firestorm has yet to subside. Critics also continue to argue that the college student subjects of the studies had not yet had enough life experiences to precipitate pathological symptoms; however, no lifetime studies have ever been done.

In 2003 meta-analysis made a repeat appearance in the *Psychological Bulletin*. Emily Ozer and colleagues at the University of California–San Francisco analyzed sixty-eight published reports looking for predictors of post-traumatic stress disorder in individuals exposed to stressful events. They found that intense negative emotions such as fear, helplessness, horror, guilt or shame, or a dissociative experience at the time of the trauma were associated with later psychopathology. Although child sexual abuse as a stressful event was not included as one of the factors in this study, the findings appear relevant.

Statistical profiles may be helpful in clarifying population patterns, but they say little or nothing about individual children at risk. The major risk factor for a child to become a victim of sexual abuse is to grow up in a family or neighborhood with an abuser in it.

The family setting most conducive to sexual abuse is one in which the male authority figure has absolute control. As previously noted, such control is often manifested by physical abuse and threats as well as emotional and sexual abuse. The rules are unpredictable and punishment for violation of them is harsh. Children are isolated from peers and threatened with terrible consequences if they reveal anything. In such a setting, children become passive and compliant and may develop a strong attachment to the abuser in an attempt to ward off attacks. It is not unusual for an older sibling to assume a powerful, sexually dominating role. The same pattern may occur in institutional settings. Low power, low status, and physically or developmentally "different" individuals in boarding schools, camps, and similar settings as well as in families may more easily become victims.

When a friend, neighbor, or extended family member is the abuser, that individual usually follows the expected modus operandi. That adult assesses potential victims for vulnerability, and the child who appears isolated or needy or particularly passive is approached first. A child with an absent parent might be at higher risk of such an approach from a trusted or respected adult but, statistically, the vast majority of victims come from intact families. The abuser first tests the potential victim with seemingly accidental touches in order to gauge the response. If the child welcomes the attention or responds passively, then the contact will increase. Such contact may occur in such a way that the abuser may continue to frame it as innocent or accidental and the victim may question his own judgment about the appropriateness of the touching. The abuser may then introduce sexual talk or pornography into the relationship and a curious, needy, or passive child may continue to go along. Eventually the abuser will find a way to be alone with the child and act out the adult's own sexual desires. A similar pattern of need and curiosity will cause children to agree to meet someone with whom they have chatted on the Internet, or to go off with a stranger.

Some pedophiles are avid users of the Internet. Pornographic pictures of children are available through file-sharing or for a price. These may be useful in developing fantasies for arousal or masturbation. Many pedophiles find validation for their interests on pedophile-oriented websites. In addition to networking with other pedophiles for files, leads, and mutual reinforcement, some use the Internet to actively seek victims. They frequent chatrooms used by children of the age and sex they prefer and gather information about particular participants. Anonymity may embolden some children and help overcome inhibitions about personal contact. Once a potential victim is identified, the pedophile may take a trust-based approach and try to build a relationship that may eventually lead to a meeting, or may solicit sex directly. Rendezvous sites are generally in neutral territory such as a motel near the child's home. The pedophile may believe that this kind of approach will avoid detection and apprehension—and they may be correct, as long as the child with whom the potential abuser exchanges sexually explicit e-mails is not an undercover police officer.

Statistical profiles of perpetrators are notoriously unreliable. The number of convictions for sexual offenses is not a good measure of their actual incidence. Most offenses go undetected, and others are plea-bargained to different, nonsexual crimes such as criminal threatening or assault. Clinical and legal samples are not representative of the population as a whole. In 1985, psychiatrist Gene Abel and colleagues published information about a unique group of offenders. These New York City men were invited to volunteer for participation in a program in which they would remain anonymous and their crimes would not be reported. They were asked to list all the sexual contacts they had ever had with children. This study could not be done today because of the requirements for mandatory reporting. Heterosexual pedophiles (not incest perpetrators) averaged 120 "completed or attempted molestations" up to that point in their lives. Homosexual pedophiles averaged 205 separate victims. Some have argued that these men were lying to impress the clinicians. However, a 1990 New Hampshire State Prison survey included incest perpetrators and the average number of lifetime victims was twenty. Three percent acknowledged more than 100 victims. In general, priests tend to have fewer victims, but some number them in the hundreds as well. Potentially, one man can do a great deal of damage, and a few molesters can put a large number of children at risk for future difficulties.

# 3. What Are the Effects of Abuse?

Survivors of rape, child sexual abuse, domestic abuse, natural disaster, terrorism, hostage-taking, and war—all situations in which a person is rendered helpless by overwhelming forces—may show the characteristic manifestations of posttraumatic stress disorder (PTSD).

The American Psychiatric Association's Diagnostic and Statistical Manual (DSM IV) identifies three clusters of symptoms that characterize PTSD: persistent reexperience of the traumatic event, persistent avoidance of stimuli associated with that trauma and numbing of general responsiveness, and persistent symptoms of increased agitation. Reexperience may be manifest as recurrent and intrusive recollections or flashbacks of the event, recurrent distressing dreams of the event, and psychological or physiological distress when exposed to internal or external cues that resemble an aspect of the traumatic event. Avoidance and numbing are seen as efforts to avoid thinking, feeling, or talking about the trauma, to avoid activities, people, or places associated with the traumatic event, and to be unable to recall certain aspects of that event. The traumatized individual shows decreased interest in significant activities, feels detached from others, and has a restricted range of affective responses and the sense of a foreshortened future. Increased arousal takes the form of difficulty in falling or staying asleep, irritability and outbursts of anger, difficulty in concentrating, hypervigilance, and an exaggerated startle response.

A diagnosis of complex post-traumatic stress disorder proposed for DSM V emphasizes that chronic abuse and abuse in childhood result in additional symptoms. These include difficulty with regulation of emotion, dissociative symptoms, and somatization or related physical complaints. Such individuals experience a damaged sense of self, chronic guilt and shame, feelings of ineffectiveness, and a chronic sense of despair and helplessness. They may idealize the perpetrator, have difficulty in establishing and maintaining trusting relationships, and display a tendency to be revictimized or to victimize others.

Harvard psychiatrist Judith Herman, M.D., summed this up by noting that such traumatic events may produce profound and lasting changes in physiologic arousal, emotion, cognition, and memory as well as in the integration of all these functions. Survivors are "disconnected from the present" and continue to react to life experiences as if they were anticipating, experiencing, or responding to the earlier trauma.

The nature and severity of symptoms may vary depending upon the age at which the trauma occurred. Younger children with fewer defenses and underdeveloped coping strategies are more susceptible to negative aftereffects and may even show significant impairment in personality development. More frequent or severe abuse, especially the trauma of penetration, sadistic abuse for the arousal of the perpetrator, extended time of abuse, a close relationship to the abuser, and the experience of multiple abusers may all increase the negative impact.

Study of the neurobiology of post-traumatic stress disorder is still in its infancy, but animal studies and limited human studies suggest that it is a discrete illness with specific physical manifestations. The human body responds and adapts to stressful events. The nervous and endocrine systems play a key role in this.

First, we need to review basic neuroanatomy. The central nervous system consists of the brain and spinal cord. The

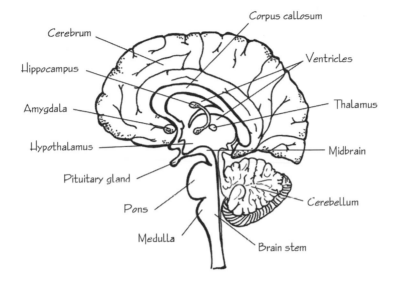

**Figure 3.1** Cross-section of Brain

peripheral nervous system carries incoming sensory input and outgoing motor responses to the rest of the body. The autonomic nervous system serves internal organs and has cells within the central nervous system. The autonomic nervous system has two parts: the sympathetic nervous system responds when the body needs to react with "fight or flight," and the parasympathetic nervous system takes over during periods of rest and restoration. The brain consists of three parts: the most primitive innermost layer, the brain stem, is responsible for basic functions such as heart rate and respiration; the central limbic system regulates affect and emotion; and the outer neocortex governs thought and language.

The neuroendocrine system sends chemical messages (hormones or neurotransmitters) to start or stop responses. The hypothalamus in the brain stem controls the endocrine glands via the pituitary gland. In response to pituitary regulation, the

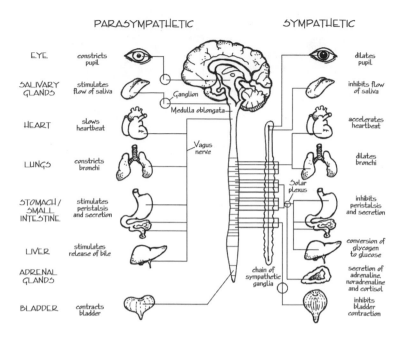

**Figure 3.2** Autonomic Nervous System

adrenal medulla (inner part) secretes the catecholamines adrenalin (epinephrine) and noradrenalin (norepinephrine) and the adrenal cortex (outer part) releases cortisol, a gluco-corticoid. The locus coeruleus (literally, "blue place") in the brain stem and sympathetic fibers themselves also produce catecholamines. Serotonin is also a catecholamine and neuro-transmitter whose role is uncertain in the stress response but appears to modulate the norepinephrine effect.

The catecholamines stimulate the sympathetic nervous system to increase heart rate, blood pressure, oxygen consumption, and blood sugar, all of which mobilize the body for action. The glucocorticoid cortisol elevates metabolism and blood sugar but also exerts negative feedback on the hypothalamus and pituitary so that a high level of cortisol closes the loop and shuts off the mobilization of catecholamines.

When a potentially stressful event occurs, the neocortex interprets and coordinates incoming stimuli and plans a response. This input is filtered by the hippocampus and amygdala. They are located in the medial temporal lobe, but are directly connected to the limbic system via the Papez circuit. The hippocampus receives the motor and sensory input and puts it into historical context. It provides relational memory and also determines if information should be stored in long-term memory or be forgotten. The amygdala assigns emotional significance to the input. The amygdala also contains many opiate and benzodiazepine receptors which, if blocked, can interfere with the conditioned emotional response. If assessment determines that "fight or flight" is indicated, the locus coeruleus releases catecholamines, the adrenal glands are stimulated via the hypothalamic-pituitary axis to release both catecholamines and glucocorticoids, and the body is activated to respond.

In most people, the stressful event ends and all these processes return to homeostatic, or balanced, baseline function. This is not true for individuals with post-traumatic stress disorder. Their systems continue to be sensitive to external stimuli and they are in a state of permanent alert, prepared for further attack. Atlanta researcher J. Douglas Bremmer, M.D., has reported changes associated with this condition in the hypothalamic-pituitary-adrenal (HPA) axis and noradrenergic systems as well as in benzodiazepine, opiate, dopaminergic and various neuropeptide systems that modulate function in the hippocampus, amygdala, and prefrontal cortex of the brain. Neuroimaging studies have shown that post-traumatic stress disorder is associated with a decrease in hippocampal volume. (It is not currently known if the hippocampus actually shrinks or if individuals susceptible to PTSD have smaller hippocampi to begin with. Neuroimaging studies have not been done on pre-morbid, asymptomatic individuals.) Without feedback about past experience and current context, the amygdala has exaggerated activation and attaches additional emotional significance to the incoming stimuli. Catecholamines are mobilized and full sympathetic arousal occurs. In individuals with post-traumatic stress disorder, cortisol is also mobilized but is quickly metabolized and does not reach a level sufficient to turn off catecholamine production. This state of hyperarousal causes hypervigilance and increased startle responses. Activation of the amygdala is associated with activity in the visual cortex that may be the basis for flashbacks and nightmares. One small aspect of the original trauma—a look, a sound, a smell, or a feeling—may trigger the whole memory picture along with all the negative emotional responses that accompanied the original event.

Boston psychiatrist Bessel Van der Kolk postulates that the extreme arousal associated with trauma floods the brain with neurotransmitters, "stamping in" vivid sensory memories of the event. These events may take the form of fragmented images that, when stimulated by present emotion, produce a vivid "reliving" of the past trauma in the present. The emotional memory system is housed in the amygdala and operates independently of cortical control. The system operates in a rapid response mode and this hypervigilance may produce sustained fear. These responses become automatic and beyond conscious control.

The overall effects may be so powerful and painful that the survivor becomes overwhelmed and cannot deal with them. Detachment, numbness, and passivity may extend to a complete denial of reality. It is not uncommon for a victim of abuse to describe the sensation of being outside the body, sometimes floating in the air, and dispassionately observing what is going on. Some theorists believe that depersonalization may progress to somatization disorder (formerly called hysteria), borderline personality disorder, and dissociative identity disorder (formerly called multiple personality disorder). The sense of disconnection may be so great that the survivor resorts to self-injury to feel something—anything. Paradoxically, the sight of one's own blood may be soothing and experienced without pain. The survivor is ultimately unable to integrate the multiple levels of response and finally assigns them to different selves rather than acknowledging that they are part of the same complex emotional reaction. Identity may be fragmented, but the individual is able to survive and to present a superficially normal façade to the world.

The world does not feel like a safe place for the sexually abused child and adult survivor. Basic trust is shattered. This is especially true when the perpetrator is a member of the family. The victim is often isolated from friends and other family members and has to deal with an often unpredictable abuser. The child may think, "Will they be angry, or drunk, or act as if I were special?" When other supposedly caring family members passively ignore—or worse, actively enable the abuse—basic trust is eroded even further. This can be devastating to potential future relationships, especially to sexual relationships. Intimacy and sexuality are often split. A survivor may want closeness but fear sexual contact and avoid both.

Debra Kalmuss, Ph.D., from the Columbia School of Public Health, defines *sexual health* as the ability to "derive pleasure from and make decisions about one's sexual and reproductive behavior and identity in a manner that respects one's own sexual rights and desires as well as those of others."

For someone on whom sex was first imposed on terms dictated by another more powerful person and not associated with pleasure, sexual health may be an unrealized dream. Sexual dysfunctions including low desire, inability to experience orgasm, vaginal muscle spasm (vaginismus), and painful intercourse are common. Sexual behavior is learned, and imposed sex is not a positive experience.

University of Nevada–Reno psychologists Leah Leonard and Victoria Follette have suggested two theories to explain the relationship between child sexual abuse and sexual dysfunction. One is experiential avoidance, a process that includes an unwillingness to reexperience painful thoughts, feelings, and memories associated with the experience of sexual abuse. The other is emotional avoidance, a process where sexual intimacy is associated with emotional pain. Both must be addressed as part of the therapeutic process.

Unwanted sexual activity may result in physical trauma, bleeding, infections, vaginal discharge, itching, urinary tract infections, abdominal pain, or pregnancy. Some clinicians have suggested that early sexual activity causes an increase in sex hormone levels, hypersexuality, and early puberty. Statistics do confirm that survivors of child sexual abuse engage in consensual sexual activity at an earlier age than do their non-abused peers. They are also less likely to use barrier forms of contraception such as condoms and are therefore more at risk of contacting sexually transmitted diseases including HIV/AIDS. They have more partners, more pregnancies, and more abortions and are more likely to be victimized in the future. Some survivors may prostitute themselves in order to have more control over who has access to their bodies and to make their partners pay for it.

Self-doubt as a result of early victimization is common. The child asks, "What did I do to deserve this?" The perpetrator often tells a female child that she is bad or just like mother and does indeed deserve the abuse. The confusion is compounded if there is any erotic aspect to the abuse, such as involuntary sexual arousal. Rewards from the abuser in the form of treats or privileges also lead to conflicting emotions. Negative feelings may make the survivor more susceptible to self-medication with drugs or alcohol, or the negativity may be converted to physical symptoms requiring relief by pre-scription medication. Self-identification as a "victim" or "damaged goods" may result in low self-esteem and create a pattern of self-destructive behavior.

Overall, the victims, and then the survivors, lose faith in what is supposed to be the natural order where children are cherished and protected, and where they are safe in the family and community. For them the world becomes unjust.

Young children who are abused may not express them-selves verbally, but may demonstrate disorganized or agitated behavior as well as highly sexualized play, inappropriate sexual knowledge, or sexually aggressive behavior. They may act out in their play what they are unable to verbalize. They may have nightmares, but these may not be specifically sexually oriented. They may regress developmentally and wet the bed, suck their fingers, or hang their heads. If the perpetrator was a stranger, the child may demonstrate separation anxiety. All are warning signs of possible abuse. Symptoms of trauma or infection would have few other explanations. Undeveloped psychological defenses and intellectual abilities make it diffi-cult for these victims to understand that they are not responsi-ble, and basic issues in trust and gender identity may be compromised.

Adolescents have multiple developmental tasks to accom-plish. They must become independent of parental control, achieve mature sexual expression, develop the capacity for intimacy and understand how it differs from sexuality, choose an adult role, and crystallize their personal value systems. Sexual abuse complicates each of these tasks. If the abuser was a parent, the conflicting feelings of attachment and hostility must be worked through or else there is great potential for future negative relationships and revictimization. Mature sexual expression gives way to aversion to sexual behavior, sexual identity confusion, and sexual dysfunction. Promiscuity—the seemingly opposite behavior—is also common. For girls, a history of sexual abuse is associated with increased teen pregnancy. Such a pregnancy is often accompanied by stress, substance abuse, and the birth of small, poorly developed babies. Teenage girls who sexually abuse younger children are likely to report a history of sexual abuse themselves. The capacity for intimacy is compromised by an inability to trust others. Adult role choices may be limited as the perception that the world is a safe place is shattered. Self-image may include worthlessness, shame, and guilt.

Any issues unresolved in adolescence will carry over into adulthood, and the resulting behavior patterns become harder to change. The intimate invasion of personal space leaves many survivors with an inability to trust other people to be close to them. The bodily invasion also seems to predispose survivors to focus on somatic responses and to develop a wide range of physical complaints. Not surprisingly, the complaints often involve lower abdominal or pelvic pain, bladder dysfunction, irritable bowel syndrome, premenstrual dysphoria, painful menstruation, chronic fatigue syndrome, and headache. It is also not surprising that women with these complaints are reluctant to seek gynecological services including Pap tests for cervical cancer screening. When they do see a physician, the often vague nature of the complaints results in a disproportionate number of surgical procedures. They may also avoid dental care.

A recent Australian study has shown that, among a group of adult women treated for depression, those with a history of child sexual abuse showed more deliberate self-harm and were more likely to have been recent victims of violence than were their depressed peers. Long-term physical consequences of abuse can become manifest in a great many ways.

According to Gelinas, low self-esteem and guilt are characteristic of the grown-up parentalized female child. These women had no rights as children and feel that they have no rights as adults. They blame themselves for being victimized and do not believe that they deserve better. (Interestingly, abused younger sisters of the parentalized child show all the traumatic effects but not the low self-esteem and guilt. They know they were not responsible.)

These women have problems with parenting; it is difficult for them to balance discipline and affection, especially after their children start to talk and make demands. Children learn to use guilt and feel entitled to have their demands met. Husbands are still needy. Often the new mother's parents continue to make demands on her as well. As she tries to deal with all these demands, she feels progressively more inadequate and withdraws. She may then begin to lean on her oldest daughter, and the cycle continues.

Such a woman may lead a life of quiet desperation until some external event triggers symptoms; promotion or selection for a position that presumes a level of competence she doesn't feel or her daughter reaching the age at which she was abused are examples. She may not demonstrate classic post-traumatic stress disorder but a disguised presentation such as chronic depression, impulsive acting out, or confusion. These women will not spontaneously report their history of abuse, and may not even realize that there is a cause-and-effect relationship. They will disclose if asked.

Progression of the psychological effects of child sexual abuse is associated with particular personality disorders. "Association" is the operative word here because, although a large number of people with these disorders report a history of child sexual abuse, many abused individuals do not develop those patterns of behavior.

Depersonalization, dissociation, and dysphoria are key elements of PTSD and are characteristic of somatization disorder, borderline personality disorder, and dissociative identity disorder as well. A person will not show all these disorders at once or sequentially, but will settle into one pattern over time.

To meet the DSM IV criteria for somatization disorder, a person must have had multiple physical symptoms beginning before age thirty and lasting a number of years. These must include pain symptoms in at least four different sites or functions, two different gastrointestinal complaints, one sexual or reproductive symptom other than pain, and one pseudoneurological symptom, none of which can be explained by a known medical condition such as an arthritic joint, an ulcer, a uterine tumor, or nerve damage.

People with borderline personality disorder have problems with relationships, self-image, affect, and impulse control. They may do anything to avoid perceived abandonment, have intense and unstable interpersonal relationships, struggle with poor self-image, feel chronically empty, demonstrate inappropriate and intense anger, and they may dissociate. Many of these symptoms are carried over from the relationship between victim and abuser.

Individuals with dissociative identity disorder take this defense to an extreme. They have two or more distinct personality states with different and enduring patterns of perceiving, relating to, and thinking about the environment and themselves. These different identities recurrently control that person's behavior, and things that happen to one identity may not be accessible to the memory of another. A history of a helpless child leaving conscious memory behind in the face of overwhelming force seems very relevant.

While the physical, sexual, and psychological consequences of child sexual abuse are generally the same for boys and girls, boys may deal with them differently. First, a boy is less likely to report abuse. If the perpetrator is female, he may not want to acknowledge that he was overpowered or controlled by a woman. He may also feel that the experience of having sex with an older woman is positive, but his subsequent behavior might indicate that this is not the case. If the perpetrator is male, the child may feel shame, embarrassment, a sense of emasculation, or the fear of being labeled as gay by others. Male anger may be expressed in acts of aggression or criminal behavior. While abused males show the same patterns of reckless and dysfunctional sexual behavior as abused females, they are more susceptible to sexual identity confusion. This is particularly so for prepubescent victims. There seems to be a statistical association between the experience of child sexual abuse and adult male homosexuality. The operative word again is association. Boys who are most attractive to male perpetrators may show effeminate behavior, lack secondary sex characteristics such as facial and pubic hair and a deepening voice, and have no peer support or strong male figures with whom to identify. These factors may contribute to a homosexual identity formation without the complicating factor of sexual abuse, but the experience of sexual activity with an older male may serve to crystallize such an identity. The same does not appear to be true for postpubescent males who may already have identified themselves as committed heterosexuals. No information is available about sexual identity distortion in girls who are abused by older women.

The effects of child sexual abuse on parenting behavior are variable. The boundary violations of abuse could result in survivors exhibiting a range of punitive, permissive, or overprotective behaviors toward their own children. They may reject or mimic their own parents' model of the parent-child relationship.

# 4. Treating the Survivor

If the worst effects of child sexual abuse are best described in terms of post-traumatic stress disorder, the best treatment approaches should follow that same paradigm. For those traumatized individuals who continue to show symptoms months or years after being abused, formal psychotherapy may offer the best chance for a better life. In general terms, the survivor (no longer a victim) must recognize the trauma, control responses to it, and integrate it into the life experience.

In her classic 1992 book *Trauma and Recovery*, Dr. Judith Herman discussed three stages of recovery from any traumatic experience: safety, remembrance and mourning, and reconnection. It is important to remember that the recovery process is not always a straight-line progression; overlap and falling back are common. Recovery cannot begin until the trauma is identified, acknowledged, and, particularly in the case of child sexual abuse, ended. Herman stresses the importance of a supporting and trusting relationship with the therapist as critical for the recovery process to take place. Telling the truth and establishing clear boundaries are integral parts of the therapeutic relationship.

Safety requires that the actual threat of danger is over and that the abuse has ended. For the abused child, this means an end to the relationship with the abuser and social support for the termination of that relationship. For the adult survivor, it means that society assigns responsibility to the abuser and harm to the victim. To restore a sense of order and justice, the perpetrator should be held legally responsible in terms of both punishment and restitution. Unfortunately, the justice system and courts do not always provide that, and the adversarial nature of the proceedings is not always a positive experience for survivors and may even lead to additional trauma. Victim advocates in the prosecutor's office and with the police can be particularly helpful in preparing and supporting survivors in dealing with a system seemingly designed to be traumatic. Cross-examination of a witness, particularly a child, can be brutal.

In addition to control of the environment, control of the body, both physical and psychological, is an integral part of safety. It is helpful at the outset for the clinician to educate the patient as to what the usual aftereffects of abuse may be. Symptoms such as hyperarousal, insomnia, or depression must be addressed specifically and directly. An overstimulated sympathetic nervous system needs to be calmed. If relaxation techniques such as biofeedback, meditation, yoga, strenuous exercise, or progressive relaxation are not effective in calming stress, then a range of medication is available to target anxiety, insomnia, depression, or other overwhelming symptoms.

Historically, physicians have prescribed sedation with alcohol, opiates, or barbiturates to deal with such symptoms; patients have also used these substances for self-medication. The results are poor because medication dependency and abuse often follow. Once it was determined that increased sympathetic arousal and increased catecholamine activity in the brain were responsible for much of the clinical picture, it became possible to utilize more specific pharmacological agents. Specific serotonin reuptake inhibitors (SSRIs), for example, reduce catecholamine levels and are now the treatment of choice. In controlled studies, SSRIs paroxetine (Paxil), sertraline (Zoloft), and fluoxetine (Prozac) produce moderate but statistically significant decreases in reexperiencing, intrusive hyperarousal, and numbing symptoms. Beta blockers such as propanolol (Inderal) and clonidine (Catapres) reduce sympathetic outflow from the central nervous system and block intrusive symptoms, especially flashbacks and nightmares.

Anticonvulsant mood stabilizers such as carbamazepine (Tegretol) reduce flashbacks and angry outbursts by blocking nerve potentiation. In severe cases, low doses of the new socalled second generation antipsychotic medications such as risperidone (Risperdal) may calm the most disturbed patients. The mechanism of action of these drugs is unknown but they are antagonists at dopamine and serotonin receptor sites. Benzodiazepine tranquilizers such as diazepam (Valium) and lorazepam (Ativan) are usually not helpful. These drugs may eliminate the symptoms temporarily, but in doing so may actually interfere with the resolution of distress and increase depression. They do not deal with the cause of the distress, only with the manifestations. Their use also raises the risk of dependence and abuse.

A few studies have been done, mostly with SSRIs, where medication was used to augment psychotherapy. Results from the combined approach are generally better than those with either one alone.

A person cannot engage in psychotherapy if the level of distress is high and the symptoms overwhelming; however, it is possible to begin the healing process by recognizing, naming, and charting the circumstances that produce symptoms and the responses to them. One can then develop plans to ensure safety and reduce distress. Some don't even require a therapist for implementation. For example, if heightened tension and insomnia are associated with the onset of darkness, then a nightlight may provide some sense of security. If panic attacks follow a walk past a perpetrator's house, then a different route home from school or a companion might be helpful.

If depression routinely follows family visits, then such visits should be modified or eliminated. Clearly it is necessary for family members and caregivers to understand and support this process so that they do not amplify the stress or even cause additional trauma to the person trying to recover. Once patterns are identified and modifications in place, the survivor has some control and responsibility for identifying the situations, behavior, or places that trigger symptomatic responses. The person then ceases to be a helpless victim, and is, instead, an active survivor.

Herman calls the second stage of recovery remembrance and mourning. Here the traumatic story is told and acknowledged to be a part of the survivor's life history. Grief for that which is lost—childhood, trust, or family—is expressed and the strong internal core of the self is validated and empowered to move on. This is the stage where psychotherapy is most helpful and it must occur in the context of a trusting therapeutic relationship.

There are often many therapists to choose from. It is always appropriate to ask a potential therapist about training, credentials, therapeutic approach, and experience with survivors of child sexual abuse. Special qualifications such as experience working with children, certification in sex therapy, or the ability to prescribe medication may be considered. It is more important to work with an experienced and trusted clinician than to take whomever the insurance panel provides. Good therapy is a solid investment in future happiness.

There is always some degree of transference in any therapeutic setting. The patient will transfer some feeling about people from the past onto the therapist. Working with those feelings is part of the therapeutic process. However, some feelings can be a barrier to treatment. If the therapist were consciously or unconsciously identified with the abuser, an enabler, an unsupportive grandparent, an aggressive police detective, or anyone else from the patient's past, that would affect the therapeutic relationship. It is essential that the patient always feel safe enough to be truthful. Similarly, the therapist may have a similar range of feelings toward the patient. This is countertransference. Seeing a patient as a whiner or as incompetent or as in need of rescue can all be problematic. Both parties in the therapeutic relationship must agree to the treatment contract: the goals, the process of achieving those goals, and the boundaries of therapy. A therapist who overidentifies with the patient as victim (especially if the therapist has a similar history of abuse), sympathizes with the perpetrator, experiences "witness guilt" or secondary trauma by listening to the patient's story, wants to rescue the patient, or considers or even experiences boundary violations in some other way should talk this through with a colleague or supervisor. The therapist is also bound to uphold his part of the treatment contract. Any therapist who works with survivors will be stressed by their histories and their pain and will need to deal with that stress response.

Experts agree that "telling the story" and coming to terms with it are essential to recovery. We know that repression is probably the most common defense mechanism used in dealing with trauma. The bad memories are pushed out of conscious awareness but continue to influence behavior. The therapist's role is to help the client deal with the past in an open-minded and supportive manner but not to direct the memory process.

Survivors are particularly adept at reading their therapists. They learned that careful attention to their abuser's statements, moods, and emotions was essential to survival and they transfer those observation skills to the therapeutic relationship. Experienced in altered states of consciousness, they may be extremely suggestible. It is therefore essential that the therapist not have preconceived notions about the origin of symptoms, as the client may pick these up. This is the basis for the repressed and recovered memory controversy.

In 1988 Ellen Bass and Laura Davis published *The Courage to Heal: A Guide for Women Survivors of Child Sexual Abuse.* They offered advice on coming to terms with known abuse but also observed that "if you are unable to remember any specific instances like the ones mentioned above but have a feeling that something abusive has happened to you, it probably did." Some therapists took this further and suggested to clients that their presenting symptoms were certainly due to child sexual abuse and then pressed them to recall the memories they had repressed. They used techniques such as hypnosis, age regression, guided fantasy, and dream interpretation. Some clients did recover memories including those of abuse in infancy. In 1991 *People* magazine published articles by comedienne Roseanne Barr Arnold and former Miss America Marilyn van Derbur detailing the memories of child sexual abuse that they had recovered. This helped open the gate, and, in pursuit of punishment and restitution, a number of civil and criminal suits were filed against alleged perpetrators as a result of recovered memories.

In a seminal article in the May 1993 *American Psychologist,* Dr. Elizabeth Loftus, then at the University of Washington and now at the University of California–Irvine, questioned "the reality of repressed memory." She pointed out that child sexual abuse was actually remembered vividly by most who reported it and that cognitive memory patterns probably did not exist before age three. Early sexual abuse provided a simple explanation for whatever problem brought the patient to therapy and this explanation was often reinforced by the therapist or by a peer group of survivors. Although these patients honestly believed that their "recovered" memories were true, Loftus pointed to many studies, including thirty years of her own research, that showed that false memories could be implanted with leading questions, suggestions, and false feedback. The subject would not only insist that the memory was real, but would also add details. Newspaper and magazine articles, reports by other victims, and suggestions may have been incorporated into the memories of a client's own "abuse." The memories were honest but false. This "false memory syndrome" was used to counter the recovered memory claim. Loftus has expressed the fear that false claims would only serve to trivialize the experiences of true victims.

As one might suppose, these divergent points of view were often argued in court with expert testimony on both sides. Judicial bodies tried to make legal sense out of conflicting claims and then issued guidelines. One representative decision was that of the New Hampshire Supreme Court in *State v. Hungerford.* Joel Hungerford's daughter had recovered memories of incest in therapy and had filed criminal charges against him. In ruling against the admission of these recovered memories, the justices wrote that the state must demonstrate "that the reasoning or methodology underlying the testimony is scientifically valid; and that it is capable of empirical testing and can properly be applied to the facts at issue." They found that it was not. They also questioned the percentage of recovered memories known to be false and noted the importance of the age of the witness at the time of the assault or assaults, the length of time between the event and the recovered memory, the presence or absence of verifiable corroborative evidence, and the circumstances of the recovery of the memory. The final point referred specifically to therapy whose purpose was to recover memory. The justices were particularly critical of therapists who ordinarily seek hidden memories, believe that many problems stem from sexual abuse, and validate allegations of abuse that do arise. As a result of this decision, Hungerford sued his daughter's therapist for damages. The suit was apparently settled out of court.

Washington, D.C., psychologist Christine Courtois developed practice guidelines for therapists of adult clients who do not initially disclose child sexual abuse. The therapist should obtain a good psychosocial history and personality assessment but not uncritically accept or confirm suspicions without corroborating evidence. The clinician should remain neutral, avoid leading questions, and remember that normal childhood memory is spotty. No symptom or set of symptoms is due exclusively to child sexual abuse and other possibilities must be considered. The clinician should keep accurate records, preface possible allegations with "the client reported" or similar words, and seek supervision for all such cases. Hypnosis is generally inappropriate, as is referral to an incest survivors group, if the client does not have conscious memory of abuse. Both have the potential for increased suggestibility. General support groups may be helpful. The therapist should not propose family confrontations or lawsuits, but should be supportive if these do occur.

The goal of treatment at this stage is to achieve an intellectual or cognitive understanding of the abuse, accept it emotionally, and change behavioral responses accordingly. Traditional individual or group psychotherapy is primarily an intellectual exercise. This therapy provides support, empathy, and the opportunity to explore the meaning of the event in the context of life experience and the inner sense of the self. The client works through and integrates the trauma so that there is no further need for maladaptive defenses.

In more active behavioral treatment, the goal is to recondition the response to trauma in order to promote change.

Through the process of *collaborative empiricism* the cognitive behavioral therapist helps the client attach the proper emotional responses to the cognitive triggers and find alternative behavioral responses to them. In *Stress and Trauma,* University of Missouri psychologist Patricia Resick describes several of the behavioral techniques that are combined with cognitive processing. In stress inoculation training, the client gradually approaches the fear-producing stimuli and extinguishes the unwanted response. The first skill taught in this and other behavioral approaches is relaxation training. In progressive muscle relaxation, the client focuses on each major muscle group of the body in turn by first tightening the muscles to help identify them and then relaxing them. The client develops a relaxing mental image to accompany the physical relaxation. With practice, the client should ultimately be able to visualize that special image, breathe out, and let go of all bodily tension. Cognitively, the client practices thought stopping. When a negative thought comes to mind, the person literally says or thinks, "Stop!", focuses on the current reality, and considers alternative ways to deal with the situation. At other times, the client practices covert rehearsal by imagining potentially fearful situations and alternative responses. The final step is to apply all of these techniques—relaxation, thought stopping, and alternative responses—in day-to-day circumstances to engage in the feared behaviors or situations. Successful engagement should be positively reinforced by acknowledgment of that success.

Exposure-based treatment may be either strictly in the imagination (covert) or done in the real world (overt). In systematic desensitization, the therapist and client together create a hierarchy of fears. In a relaxed state, the client imagines a situation briefly and repetitively and then relaxes as soon as a fear or anxiety is experienced. By backing off and then approaching again, the client should be able to advance through the hierarchy. The well-rehearsed relaxed response should then be transferable to the real world. In "flooding," the client combines relaxation with the experience of prolonged, real exposure to fear-producing cues. Distress should decrease with each subsequent exposure as the client realizes that nothing bad has happened as a result of that exposure.

These behavioral techniques are combined with cognitive processing. This goes beyond the raw emotional response to the trauma and explores the distorted thinking that has resulted. False beliefs such as "I brought it on myself" or "I should have stopped him" need to be addressed as well.

Trauma-focused cognitive behavioral therapy is particularly helpful for children. One study compared child-centered therapy where abused children talked about trauma at their own pace with trauma-focused cognitive behavioral therapy. In addition to the first group's trying to make sense of the experience and identify more effective future responses, a second group of abused children was encouraged to confront increasingly detailed and distressing abuse-related reminders and memories. This was done in a way that was comfortable for each child. Choosing a method of exposure such as imagery, doll play, drawing, reading, letter writing, poetry, or singing gave each child more sense of control. The children kept journals and discussed them with their non-abusing caregivers. The second group did twice as well as the first at resolving symptoms including depression, behavioral problems, and feelings of shame.

For the therapist dealing with a trauma survivor who was a parentalized child, it is important to remember that despite the abuse, parental loyalty is still strong. The suggestion of early, direct confrontation with the abuser may drive the client away. It is more productive to focus on the illegitimacy of the behavior, its exploitive nature, and the responsibility of the abuser. It is not productive to stress the illegality of the behavior; the survivor may still be protective of abusive parents, and prosecution is impossible anyway if the statute of limitations has expired. Once the survivor is engaged in therapy, it may then be possible to deal more effectively with parents who may still be making demands on the child whom they abused. It is not helpful to blame a mother for initiating the process if she was a victim of abuse herself.

It is important to continue to address physiological disturbances of post-traumatic stress that interfere with the ability to engage in therapy. While some clinicians would address specific symptoms such as anxiety, insomnia, nightmares, flashbacks, eating disorders, headaches, pelvic pain, or chronic fatigue pharmacologically, others would consider them all to be manifestations of post-traumatic neurobiological deregulation and seek to address them more generally.

One such general approach is called eye movement desensitization and reprocessing, or EMDR. This treatment format was developed by Francine Shapiro, Ph.D., and first published in 1989. Shapiro believes that traumatic experiences leave unprocessed perceptions and that these may be resolved through the accelerated information processing that is EMDR. The clinical protocol involves eight stages that include history taking, client preparation, target assessment, desensitization, installation, body scan, closure, and reevaluation of treatment effects. The therapy itself has no empirical basis other than the observation that the stage of rapid eye movement (REM) sleep is associated with vivid dreams but physical relaxation. More intense negative emotion is correlated with more rapid eye movement. The client is encouraged to visualize the targeted image, rehearse positive thoughts, monitor physical distress and follow the therapist's finger as it moves across the visual field twice per second for twenty-four repetitions. The client then relaxes and scores the episode. It is important to be able to quantify both the intensity of the image and the degree of distress. A ten-point scale, often in terms of how full a container might be, is used. The client learns to pair a positive statement with the negative image, such as "It hurt but I survived." Over repeated exposure, high-scoring negative images accompanied by positive statements should produce lower scores in disturbance, or more relaxation. The process provides a rapid learning experience where new skills and adaptive behaviors replace dysfunctional ones. The patient is no longer stuck in old patterns and is now able to work through the feeling process.

Proponents hypothesize that the positive and negative aspects of right and left brain function become synchronized and negative cognitions become associated with positive emotions. EMDR practitioners acknowledge that their therapy does not work for everyone, but they believe it can be an effective tool in the therapeutic arsenal. Critics argue that it is simply a new twist on systematic desensitization through repeated exposure. Controlled studies have also suggested that the lateral eye movements are not necessary for improvement; benefits may be an example of client suggestibility.

Other treatment approaches, such as acupuncture and body-work to free up "muscle memories," have been suggested; anecdotal evidence exists of success with some people, but these approaches have not been subjected to rigorous evaluation.

When a person loses a part of himself, even a negative part such as a dysfunctional behavior, there is grief work to be done. Something has been lost, even if the inner self has been healed. Neurophysiologic symptoms are gone, but so are general fantasies of basic trust, idealized good parents, and a happy childhood. All must be mourned and put to rest.

A person must also accept that it may be too late to get even in terms of punishment or compensation. Anger at parents, school, church, social service agencies, police, or whoever else did not protect and defend the victim is understandable but counterproductive.

Herman's third stage of recovery is reconnection. Here the recovering survivor achieves a different view of the world and his or her place in it. There is now a future to look forward to. Reconnection with other people begins, but sexual intimacy is often the most difficult part of connection to achieve. Most survivors need a patient partner and often a good sex therapist to gradually regain or find the level of trust that will enable them to enjoy sexual desire and orgasm. A certified sex therapist has many hours of training and supervision and is recognized as such by the American Association of Sex Educators, Counselors, and Therapists. The therapist must not push the client into the more traditional sex therapy exercises such as massage because that will only increase resistance. Oregon social worker Wendy Maltz has suggested a number of touch exercises that may be more appropriate for resistant survivors. These include touching a variety of sensual objects in a basket, clapping hands with the partner, writing letters on the partner's back with a finger, creating a safe "nest" for calm nonsexual touch and having a clear system of signals for controlling touch. In these exercises, the survivor feels safe, has time to deal with associated negative images, and maintains emotional intimacy as sexual stimulation increases.

A survivor might seek personal empowerment through training in self-defense, sport, or a wilderness experience where danger is faced and overcome and survival acknowledged. Confrontation of offending or collaborating family members might be carefully considered, but only in the context of empowerment and not with an expectation of remorse or apology. Desecration of a grave may offer some sense of closure but obviously is not going to affect a deceased perpetrator.

Survivor groups can provide mutual support and engage in the mission of making the public more aware of child sexual abuse and its aftereffects. A support group can also be extremely helpful in dealing with regressions that inevitably occur.

Recovery is never truly complete; seemingly unrelated events are stressful and may revive old feelings and symptoms that had been successfully resolved. Changes in physical health and interpersonal relationships are part of life. Uterine cancer, death of a parent, or birth of a child are obvious stressors—but so are promotions, children starting school, and the death of a pet. Stress happens and must be conquered again and again.

Post-traumatic growth is a relatively recent concept. University of North Carolina psychologists Richard Tedeschi and Lawrence Calhoun have reported positive changes that may result from trauma. These include improved relationships, new possibilities for one's life, a greater appreciation for life, and a greater sense of personal strength and spiritual development. Survivors may be more vulnerable, but they are also more sure of their own capacity to survive and prevail. They acknowledge that life circumstances have changed; they are able to adapt and are more emotionally engaged and attuned to existential and spiritual matters. This positive concept does not minimize the impact of trauma but provides hope for a better life ahead.

# 5. Treating the Abuser

"Lock him up and throw away the key." "Castrate him." The former punishment for sexual offenders is practiced in "three strikes and you're out" jurisdictions after a third conviction; the latter is practiced in some Eastern European countries. One takes away access to potential victims; the other takes away desire for sex and the ability to perform. The vast majority of sexual abusers experience neither life in prison nor castration, but society demands that something be done to ensure public safety. Courts order that perpetrators be treated and sometimes even order that they be declared "cured" or "safe" before they can be released. Sex-offender treatment programs respond to that demand. Most operate on a solid theoretical base, but the question remains: do they make any difference?

In 1985 psychiatrist Gene Abel, then at Columbia University, outlined a treatment approach that encompassed five strategies: correct cognitive distortions, provide sex education, promote social skills, decrease deviant arousal, and increase nondeviant arousal. All treatment programs include these strategies, although not necessarily in those terms or with equal emphasis.

Sex offenders often see the world through different eyes. Sex-starved nine-year-old girls jump out of the bushes to attack unsuspecting men; men who touch young boys provide them with an education about how the body works; kids consent to have sex with adults; no harm comes from touching or being touched; daughters should submit to fathers' demands. All these beliefs are wrong, but offenders believe them to be true. Such distorted views must be addressed.

As a group, sex offenders may know less about sex than most people do. They may avoid adult sexual relationships for fear of appearing inadequate or they may really be inadequate. They may often be unaware of the dangers of unprotected sex and not consider the possibility of sexually transmitted diseases or unwanted pregnancy, especially with activity other than vaginal penetration. They may have a lot to learn.

Offenders tend to lack appropriate social skills. They may know how to tempt or threaten a child but are unable to approach an adult to establish a relationship that could potentially become a sexual one. More important, they lack the tools to deal effectively with strong emotions such as anger or a need for comfort and support. They have not been socialized appropriately and need such training.

Deviant arousal patterns need to be extinguished, but first they need to be identified. Certain stimuli, emotions, or circumstances are associated with episodes of abuse. A pornographic video, intoxication, and access are simple examples; however, the scenario preceding sexual acting-out is usually more complex. If there is confirmed arousal to inappropriate stimuli, measures may need to be taken to extinguish it. Potentially, these measures can be quite punitive.

The strategy most difficult to implement is increasing arousal to nondeviant stimuli. A man aroused by the sight of a scantily clad adult of the opposite sex would have a hard time being reconditioned to arousal by being urinated on, viewing a corpse, or whipping someone. Similarly, a man turned on by a prepubescent boy would have difficulty being reconditioned to arousal by the sight of a scantily clad woman. An individual may not be able to change an arousal pattern but can learn not to act on the inappropriate desire it evokes.

Treatment programs employ these strategies in different ways. Almost all occur in a correctional setting after the abuser has been caught, convicted, and sentenced. Rarely does an individual volunteer that he is abusing a child or children, because that is a reportable offense in all jurisdictions. Such an admission is most probably a call for help and should be taken seriously. While some therapists feel that they can counsel sex offenders one-on-one, they are susceptible to lies, half-truths, and distortions and may be overly invested in seeing themselves as successful. The most effective treatment venue is the therapeutic community with its emphasis on group interaction. No one understands an offender's con games better than another offender.

A therapeutic community is a highly structured environment where people work together to help themselves and each other. Punishment and privileges are determined by group consensus and peer pressure is important in fostering change. A program typically lasts for several months, with multiple opportunities to observe the progress of other offenders in the program.

Most programs have selective criteria for admission. These generally include a commitment to long-term treatment, adjustment within the institution, absence of severe psychopathology, recognition of the severity of the problem, and, most important, full and open admission that everything the victim said and for which he was convicted was true. Denial is cause for exclusion—even though there is no objective evidence that such denial has any bearing on the treatment outcome or recidivism rate. It may make the therapist and especially the prosecutor feel better if the prisoner acknowledges guilt, but the incest perpetrator who denies that he penetrated his daughter may still have a better prognosis than the serial pedophile who cheerfully admits raping twenty boys.

Prisoners are usually highly motivated to seek therapy. It may be a requirement for early release. Child molesters are on the lowest rung of the prisoner hierarchy and are often abused themselves in a general prison population. Failure to be selected for treatment means longer and harder time.

The first step in most programs is a treatment contract where the offender agrees to abide by the rules and makes a commitment to behavioral change. Failure to progress in treatment or infractions of institutional or unit rules will result in termination. A psychosocial history and psychological assessment will be completed. At this time, two physiologic measures may be introduced: the polygraph and the penile plethysmograph. The polygraph, or lie detector, does not really detect lies. It detects fear by measuring the physiologic reactions associated with autonomic nervous system arousal. These are increased heart rate, rapid breathing, and sweating of the palms. The measure is used primarily to assess the level of internal response to the denial of guilt in specific offenses and in assessing the validity of the overall history of offenses.

The penile plethysmograph, or phallometer or "peter meter," directly measures penile tumescence (erection) with a strain gauge in response to a range of visual and auditory stimuli. Arousal to standardized slides of a variety of subjects, male and female, young and old, in sexual situations portraying degrees of force and seduction are compared with responses to pictures of consensual sexual activity between adults and neutral controls such as landscapes. Results are helpful in confirming or denying the true objects of arousal, and serial testing can monitor progress within the program. Neither the polygraph nor the plethysmograph has enough validity to be used in court, but they can be helpful in the treatment process once concerns about informed consent and self-incrimination have been resolved.

The first treatment phase focuses on group process and individual awareness as to why the offense occurred. A review of the four factors and a determination of how they apply to each offender are common. The effects of abuse are made clear with videos and discussions about trauma and often with confrontation by adult survivors of abuse who tell about their own life experiences. Specific groups may address issues peculiar to offenders who were themselves abused as children or who need particular help with acquiring social skills. Self-help groups such as Alcoholics Anonymous or Narcotics Anonymous may also be appropriate, as may Sex Addicts Anonymous. Offenders engage in discussion groups based on relevant books such as *Out of the Shadows* by Patrick Carnes or the sex-offender workbook series developed by William Pithers. The "sex addict" model espoused here must not be allowed to serve as a rationalization for bad behavior, but must rather be a format for behavioral change. Dr. John Bancroft at the Kinsey Institute has cautioned that terms like "sexual addiction" and "compulsive sexual behavior" are misleading because out-of-control sexual behavior has multiple causes. It is often associated with short-term mood disturbance, and the problem of clinical depression should be addressed in these cases.

Specific pharmacologic interventions may occur at this time. The anticonvulsant carbamazepine (Tegretol) may reduce impulsivity. A long-acting benzodiazepine tranquilizer such as clonazepam (Klonopin) may be used to reduce chronic anxiety. There is a high rate of depression among offenders and studies have shown this to be a comorbid condition rather than the result of incarceration. Appropriate antidepressant therapy may be indicated. As noted, the concept of "sexual compulsivity" is a controversial one; however, if there is a driven element to the sexual behavior, medications such as specific serotonin reuptake inhibitors (Prozac, Zoloft, or Paxil) may be helpful. Studies have shown that increasing central serotonin levels does reduce a high sex drive in rats and mice. As is the case with survivors, it is difficult to engage offenders in the treatment process as long as they remain focused on symptoms. Relief of these symptoms promotes that engagement.

The second phase is a continuation of the first augmented by specific group therapy experiences such as anger management, self-esteem development, stress management, or sex education and awareness. Individual work may target specific patterns of arousal. The offender may be asked to keep a "fantasy diary" to monitor his sexual thoughts. Various behavioral techniques are then utilized to extinguish deviant fantasies. Covert sensitization is an internal mental process that pairs a deviant sexual fantasy with an image such as arrest or public humiliation. Aversive conditioning pairs the fantasy with an actual noxious stimulus. Rotten meat and ammonia seem to be favorites, but electric shock has also been employed. Ideally, the diary should document a decreasing frequency of potentially troublesome fantasies and the plethysmograph should confirm this.

A somewhat more controversial technique is known as masturbatory satiation. The individual is asked to masturbate quickly to orgasm and then to continue to masturbate for twenty or thirty minutes to his favorite deviant fantasy. Normally, there is a refractory period after one orgasm before a man can have another. Trying to satisfy the fantasy with a nonresponsive penis should extinguish the power of the fantasy. One potential problem with this technique is that, in a young, multi-orgasmic man, it might actually reinforce that fantasy. Another problem is keeping the individual on track with his fantasy. This is best done by ongoing tape recording of fantasies in each practice session. Someone must then monitor the tapes to ensure compliance.

Masturbation is also suggested as a way to increase nondeviant arousal. A positive scenario involving consenting adults is developed and rehearsed. The individual then masturbates to orgasm with that scenario in mind. That should also be monitored carefully by audiotape, as there is a good deal of room for deception in reporting the actual content of the fantasy.

When behavioral treatment fails, medication may be introduced. Medroxyprogesterone acetate (Depo-Provera) and Cyproterone acetate (not currently approved for use in the United States) are anti-androgens; they lower testosterone levels by inhibiting gonadotropin secretion. The result is "chemical castration," as testosterone is required for both sexual arousal and sexual performance. Men with very low testosterone levels have no desire for sex and no erections. Use of these medications interferes with the monitoring of arousal patterns, and the effect lasts only as long as the medication is used because these drugs do not affect the body's ability to synthesize new testosterone.

Family therapy may also be introduced at this phase. Family members may participate in separate groups in order to understand offender dynamics, learn to protect children, and provide mutual support. Couples therapy may help improve communication or address specific family dynamics or sexual dysfunctions.

In the third phase of treatment, the offender continues his own work and may mentor new arrivals in the therapeutic community and lead some of the self-help groups. Emphasis turns to healthy relationships and relapse prevention. The individual must recognize the thoughts, feelings, and situations that contribute to offending behaviors and learn how to intervene at the earliest possible point in his cycle. He does this by rehearsing alternative, more socially appropriate responses.

At the conclusion of this treatment phase the abuser should accept full responsibility for his behavior, be able to recite the cycle of thoughts, feelings, and behaviors that precede offenses, be able to quickly control the deviant urges, and recognize the need for ongoing treatment in the general prison population or in the community at large.

The prediction of success or failure at the end of a treatment program is an inexact science. Abusers inevitably report themselves cured and promise never to offend again. Therapists try to be more objective, but each has an unconscious tendency to believe that his success rate is better than anyone else's. Belief in success probably helps prevent burnout in dealing with this extremely difficult population. Ongoing training and support is essential for any therapist who works with such a high-risk group.

A number of scales have been developed to try to make an objective assessment of potential dangerousness. These range from simple questionnaires to extensive computer-scored assessments. The least valid are those that include offender self-evaluation; after any treatment program, an offender will know what responses are socially desirable and answer accordingly. From an actuarial perspective, history is an excellent predictor of future offenses. Recidivism is most associated with offenders who have had a male victim, a younger victim, multiple victims, and extrafamilial victims. Sadistic sexual behavior in the past, pro-offending attitudes, and a lack of intimate relationships are also associated with re-offending. The single best predictor is continued arousal to children as measured by the penile plethysmograph. Sophisticated offenders can fake interest in other subjects because no one else really knows what they are fantasizing to the picture on the screen; however, continued arousal after completion of a treatment program is not a positive outcome. The final report should be as objective as possible, and success is always conditional. If the thoughts, feelings, or circumstances that trigger an offense are no longer controlled, the danger of an inappropriate sexual response is greater.

As previously noted, the treatment model has a solid theoretical base but the question remains: does treatment work? The short answer is, probably not. The rate of re-offending for treated and untreated groups seems to be about the same. The man who fondled a particular child when intoxicated will probably not re-offend if he stays sober, access to that child has been terminated, and he does not want to repeat the prison experience. He may now understand everything about the dynamics of his behavior, but this person was not going to re-offend anyway. On the other hand, the serial pedophile may learn to say all the right things during the treatment program but not change his behavior.

A 2004 Canadian study compared the recidivism rate of 321 untreated offenders with that of 403 who had undergone treatment over a twelve-year period. One in five in each group re-offended. Twenty percent does seem to be the generally acknowledged rate of recidivism for sex offenders. Considering that completion of a sex-offender treatment program may take years off a prison sentence, treatment may actually increase the risk to the public by releasing offenders too early.

Despite the depressing statistics, it is unlikely that programs will change anytime soon. Prosecutors and defense attorneys want them to exist. If the accused could not plea-bargain for treatment, there would be even more trials in an already overburdened court system. Sex-offender treatment is a growth industry; many therapists and institutions have a vested interest in its continuation. Sex-offender treatment is not the only modality of unproven value to enjoy popular support (Drug Abuse Resistance Education and abstinence-only sex education come immediately to mind). Perhaps those third-strike and Eastern European courts have the solution after all. The recidivism rate for those serving life sentences is zero and between 1 and 10 percent for those who have been castrated.

Realistically, then, it is extremely difficult to alter the arousal patterns of a pedophile. Of the four factors identified by the Finkelhor group, sexual arousal and emotional congruence are products of early childhood experience and are part of who the person is. By addressing issues of blockage and disinhibition, the therapist may modulate the response to sexual desire; however, because circumstances change, there are no guarantees to future control of acting-out behavior. As Boyle quotes one man on completion of a correctional treatment program: "I wasn't convinced it was wrong; I was convinced I shouldn't do it." This man, and others like him, should never be alone with a child again.

# 6. Prevention

Primary prevention is the ideal result of any intervention in a pathological process. The preventive model of public health was developed with reference to infectious diseases and is most easily applied to them. In primary prevention, a healthy person does not contract the disease. Immunization against smallpox and mosquito control to eliminate yellow fever are examples of primary prevention. In secondary prevention, a person may be asymptomatic but have disease risk factors or preclinical disease. Pap smears for cervical cancer, PSA screening for prostate cancer, and weight control and smoking cessation where there is a strong family history of heart disease are all measures that allow early intervention should an existing disease be discovered, and then allow time for effective treatment. Tertiary preventive measures take place after a person shows signs or symptoms of illness but before secondary problems have occurred. Debriding a wound to prevent gangrene or treating AIDS to prevent a viral or fungal superinfection accomplish this.

The preventive model is more difficult to apply to post-traumatic stress disorders, including those caused by childhood sexual abuse. In an ideal world, trauma would be eliminated. If children were made aware of the danger and internalized such devices as "recognize, resist, and report" or "say 'no' and tell someone" when confronted with a high-risk situation, those measures would prevent the trauma and, by extension, prevent post-traumatic stress disorder. If researchers could study resilient survivors and determine whether they possess teachable skills, then the teaching of those skills could prevent disorder from occurring after a traumatic experience. It is impossible to identify potential offenders before they decide to offend. Society cannot lock up everyone who fits the profile of a pedophile or incest perpetrator. Locking up repeat offenders who might abuse children, who would then grow up to abuse other children, could be considered primary prevention for that second generation of offenders. At this point in time there is no way to inoculate against child sexual abuse.

Secondary prevention is also difficult. A registry of known sex offenders might be considered helpful for families with children at risk in order to identify potential assailants and therefore avoid abuse. People are generally healthy before a traumatic event so there is no preclinical sign like an abnormal Pap smear to encourage early intervention; however, knowing the characteristics of those most likely to develop symptoms of PTSD after trauma might encourage such intervention. Debriefing or talking through a traumatic experience may be marginally helpful after mass disasters, but is not applicable to child sexual abuse. Some clinicians might argue that recovering memories of abuse and dealing with them after a person comes to therapy for nonspecific symptoms such as depression or weight gain would represent secondary prevention, but that intervention is controversial at best. Similarly, it is difficult to identify individuals who are at high risk of offending and encourage them to resist the urges. Addressing disinhibiting factors, such as alcohol and drug consumption or stress in individuals with other factors that might lead to child sexual abuse, would be preventive. One group trying to reach potential offenders is called Stop It Now. This group has hotlines in several cities. An individual who feels the urge to offend can call in and be referred to appropriate services to prevent his acting out. One drawback to this approach is that the hotline is legally obligated to report offenses that have already occurred. Another example of early intervention is the police "sting" operation where an officer poses as a child on the Internet. When the potential perpetrator tries to meet the "child," he is arrested. Communications leading up to such an arrest must be carefully documented in order to avoid a defense of entrapment.

Psychotherapists provide tertiary interventions. A client presents with symptoms of post-traumatic stress and seeks relief from further deterioration or new symptoms. Identified abusers may seek interventions that will prevent future episodes or worse consequences.

Some interventions may serve to facilitate more than one level of prevention. Incarceration (primary) or treatment (tertiary) of an offender may spare a person at risk (secondary) from committing further abuses.

Despite the fact that fewer than 10 percent of child molesters are unknown to their victims, the principal focus of most abuse prevention efforts is the recognition of "stranger danger." A typical set of rules to teach a child is posted on the California Attorney General's website: "Stay away from people who call you near their car; If someone tries to take you away, yell 'This person is not my father (or mother)' and scream; If you get lost in a store, find another mom with children or go to the checkout counter; Don't keep secrets from your parents; No one should touch you in parts covered by your bathing suit and you shouldn't be asked to touch anyone there either; Don't let anyone take your picture without permission from your parents or teacher."

The most important advice, however, is for parents to "help protect your child by establishing a home environment where your child feels safe to tell you anything, without fear of shame, ridicule, or punishment." This advice is echoed by the New Hampshire Coalition Against Domestic and Sexual

Violence: "Make sure your child knows that their body is their own and no one should do anything to it that makes them feel uncomfortable, sad, or bad. They have a right to say 'no' if someone tries to touch them and not keep it a secret. If a secret makes a child feel sad, bad, or afraid, it is a secret they should not keep."

This is good advice and obviously applicable in situations where the potential or actual abuser is not a stranger; however, it is not advice that is readily available. If one thought that recognition and prevention of sexual abuse were a job for the schools, one would be mistaken. Although there certainly are exceptions, teachers, as a rule, do not talk about sex or sexual abuse. They are not trained to do so, are uncomfortable with the subject, and think it is a parental responsibility. Parents don't want teachers to talk about sex, are not trained to do so themselves, and are uncomfortable with the subject. Many teachers have a standard response to tough questions: "That's a very good question but you should ask your parents when you get home. We need to get on with the lesson for today." Chances are, that will be the end of the query.

Two organizations do have active programs in sexual abuse prevention. Such programs are aimed at protecting children, adults, and the organizations themselves. The Catholic Church and the Boy Scouts of America have much to be concerned about in this regard; both face multiple lawsuits for failure to protect children.

The Catholic Church now requires all adults, including volunteers, who work with children to take youth protection training. One commonly used program is "Protecting God's Children." Formal classroom training is followed by required online testing. After completing the program, a person should recognize the warning signs that an adult may wish to perpetrate abuse, know how to control who has access to children, know how to monitor programs that involve children, be aware of changes in childhood behavior that may signal abuse, and know the procedures for communicating concern to the appropriate authority.

The program warns participants to pay particular attention to adults who prefer to spend time and form friendships with children, try to spend time with them alone, touch too much, give special gifts, and have a "favorite" child or children. These individuals bend the rules with children and discourage other adults from participating. They may use inappropriate language, tell dirty jokes, and show pornography to children.

When hiring or recruiting adults who are to have access to children, supervisors should check references and previous employers, obtain criminal background checks, and stress zero tolerance for unsafe behavior. Some dioceses exclude individuals with speeding tickets or other moving motor vehicle violations as potentially dangerous. Programs should be monitored so that adults can always be observed if not overheard when with children. Any secluded areas or unused rooms should be secured. More than one adult should always be involved in a program; parental visits and spot checks by supervisors are encouraged.

Persons responsible for the care of children should know these children well enough that any sudden changes in behavior, personal care, or relationships would be recognized. Concerns about suspicious or inappropriate behavior by either children or adults should be reported within the church chain of command and to the appropriate civil authority.

The Church has also prepared materials for parents and urges them to start early in identifying "teachable moments" to talk to their children about sex and sexual abuse so that the children will then be comfortable in talking to the parents about inappropriate touches or bad feelings about secrets. Children should rehearse saying "no" in these circumstances and know how to contact a safe person at these times.

An audiovisual part of the training does point out that priests, too, can abuse children. That warning is not included in the written handouts. The Church does appear committed to removing abusive priests from the ministry and did remove about seven hundred in the two years 2002 and 2003. Part of that commitment is also due to multimillion-dollar settlements with victims. These have resulted in curtailment of other services, closing of parishes, and, in at least three cases, bankruptcy of a diocese.

The Boy Scouts of America (BSA) also has a course in Youth Protection that is required of all summer camp staff and adult volunteers. Concern about harm caused to children by abuse, the effect of abuse on the reputation of the BSA in terms of membership and community support, millions of dollars in settlements, and the subsequent effect on the BSA's liability insurance program are all factors in this requirement. Escalating insurance premiums effect programs and have resulted in liability surcharges on the annual registration fees of both individuals and units. New volunteers are now required to undergo criminal background checks and names are checked against the confidential file.

The program content of Boy Scout training is similar to that of Church training. The Scouts have also produced the videos *It Happened to Me* for six- to nine-year-olds and *A Time to Tell* for eleven- to thirteen-year-olds to educate youth about sexual abuse. Examples of abusers on the videos include a cousin, a neighbor, and a coach, but not a Scout leader. The Scouts suggest that young boys should see the video with their parents. As an alternative, they recommend that parents review the videos before they are shown to boys because it is important for parents to be supportive, not to blame the child, and to clearly assign responsibility to the perpetrator. BSA policy now requires that two adults always be present at any Scout activity and that an adult not be alone with a child, especially on camping trips. All incidents and suspicions should be reported to Boy Scout authorities.

The current *Boy Scout Handbook* now contains a section on sexual abuse. "You do not have to let people touch you in ways you find uncomfortable. If you are ever asked to do something you know is wrong, you have the right to refuse." It goes on to stress the "three R's" of Recognize, Resist, and Report. The handbook also includes a tear-out parents' supplement that cites a few more statistics about sexual abuse, lists some possible warning signs, and encourages parents to keep talking to their children. The BSA has yet to address the problem that those individuals who work closely with the boys are generally recruited by the parents of those boys. Busy parents are unlikely to check the references of a potential volunteer and that screening is left to the formal registration process.

In 1994, seven-year-old Megan Kanka of Hamilton Township, New Jersey, was raped and murdered by a man who had recently moved in across the street. Jesse Timmendequas had two prior convictions for child molestation but the Kanka family was unaware of his history. As a result of this tragedy, in 1996 Congress passed and President Clinton signed "Megan's Law," requiring each state to develop and make available to the public a registry of known sex offenders in the community. The legislation gave states discretion in establishing criteria for disclosure but compelled them to make the information public. The New Jersey criteria are typical for registration of "sex offenders and offenders who commit predatory acts upon children." A person convicted (adult), adjudicated delinquent (juvenile), or found not guilty by reason of insanity in the commission of a sex offense is required to register with the Office of the Attorney General when he is released, moves into the state, or changes addresses within the state. New Jersey recognized three levels of risk and notification: 1) the local police, 2) local police plus schools and religious and youth organizations, and 3) the general public. An offender can petition to terminate his registration after fifteen years without incident.

Every state now has some version of Megan's Law. Access to the Sex Offender Registry varies widely. In some states the public must visit the local police station to look at the list or call a specific hotline, which may not be toll-free. Other states post some or all names and addresses of registrants on the Internet. These laws have been challenged on a number of points, but in 2002 the United States Supreme Court handed down two decisions that affirmed their existence. In *Smith v. Doe*, an Alaska case, the Court ruled that "ex-post facto" registration was not "double jeopardy" and did not extend a sentence that had already been completed because registration was "non-punitive." Since the registry stated that known offenders were not supposed to be harassed in the community, they were not being punished. In *Connecticut Department of Public Safety v. Doe*, the Court ruled that registration is not a deprivation of liberty and that an individual assessment of current danger is not necessary prior to registration.

In August 2004, Massachusetts became the forty-third state to post the names, addresses, and photos of registered offenders on the Internet. Such posting is limited to so-called Level 3 offenders where "danger to the public is high and the individual is likely to reoffend." In ruling on the challenge that posting this information would make the identified individuals subject to vigilante justice, solicitation by pornographers and other sex offenders, and complicate rehabilitation and reintegration into society, the Massachusetts Supreme Judicial Court ruled that "this is not a utopian society" and the posting served to protect society at large.

Critics continue to point out that since the vast majority of offenders are already known to the family, these lists serve no useful purpose. Even advocates of posting agree that only the most potentially dangerous offenders should be listed because there would otherwise be a flood of information. There are 18,000 registered offenders in Massachusetts alone, but only 975 names were initially posted on the Internet. The controversy will continue as some states seek to add workplace information to the name, address, and photo already posted. Some people see a sort of poetic justice in the fact that pedophiles who solicited sex on the Internet may now find their own photo posted there. They may even be able to register as a sex offender online. The major limitation to any form of listing, however, is that a concerned parent must check repeatedly to see if someone on the list might have recently moved into the neighborhood.

In addition to posting names and addresses, Massachusetts will also use global positioning systems (GPS) and electronic bracelets to track sex offenders still on probation or parole. The GPS device will enable authorities to locate the offender within ten yards of his position and will also signal if it has been removed. Proponents argue that such tracking will not only make the public safer, but will protect the offender from suspicion should an incident occur in his neighborhood. Proposals to extend the monitoring program to those offenders who have completed court supervision would certainly be subject to constitutional challenge.

While primary prevention remains the goal, it is currently an elusive one. Early intervention and effective treatment remain the best hope for protecting children, decreasing disability, and maintaining personal freedom. Researchers continue to pursue earlier and earlier markers of deviation and vulnerability in the hope that they might someday make a true breakthrough in preventive medicine.

# 7. The Search for Answers

Women who have been sexually abused as children are more likely to breast-feed their own children than are women who were not abused. Pedophiles are more likely to report head trauma before age thirteen than are all people in the general population. What is the significance, if any, of these observations? One man who fantasizes exclusively about preadolescent boys has no contact with them but writes a story about a boy who never grows up. Another volunteers to be a Little League coach in order to be in a position to maneuver boys to his home. How are they different? One child who has sexual contact with an adult is psychologically devastated, another shrugs it off, and a third thinks it was a wonderful experience. How can there be such a wide range of reactions? Research interest in the aftereffects of adult-child sex has increased dramatically in recent years, but questions remain in every aspect of this problem area.

The scope of the problem is the first concern. Standardization of the definition of child sexual abuse would be a good first step. Age, age differential, type of contact, and perceived harm are all important variables. Studies of people in therapy or in prison have selection bias and are not representative of the population as a whole. When the general population is surveyed, the methodology is not standardized. Critical data on racial and ethnic groups with regard to incidence and personal and community aftereffects are woefully inadequate. This is true for the United States and for other countries as well. Are there particular demographic or personal or community dynamics associated with seemingly high-risk groups such as Catholic priests? The duty to report child abuse limits the ability of researchers to obtain honest historical data. It is impossible to identify the so-called non-contact pedophiles who are aroused by children but do not act out. They are a group that requires further study.

Memory is another concern. The battle between "repressed memory" advocates and "false memory" advocates continues unabated. While "false memory" researchers design studies that new "memories" can, in fact, be implanted, the "repressed memory" group continues to pile up anecdotal evidence that their clients are recovering memories of the true past. It may not be good science, but it is somehow comforting to have an explanation for a problem.

The treatment of both victims and perpetrators is fraught with potential ethical dilemmas. It is sometimes difficult to establish that patients or inmates have given truly informed consent when therapeutic intervention is recommended. A complete and documented explanation of potential risks and benefits is often irrelevant to someone wanting to get better or get out. There is also another ethical dilemma in withholding therapy that has been shown to be beneficial. There are not many randomly assigned, double-blind crossover studies in the pharmacologic treatment of post-traumatic stress disorder. "Control" subjects on a waiting list must ultimately be offered treatment.

## For Survivors

With regard to psychotherapeutic interventions, there are a limited number of outcome studies; those that have been done usually have only a three- or six-month followup. Long-term followup is a time-consuming and expensive process, but it must be done in order to determine, for example, if psychotherapy, cognitive behavioral therapy, or EMDR produces long-lasting results. If all are equally beneficial in the short term because of the positive relationship with a therapist of any of these orientations, then what is the basis for choosing one treatment over another? What results should clients and insurers demand for their healthcare dollar?

Not everyone who is traumatized develops pathological symptoms. It is important to understand why some people are resilient to stress and others thrive on it. Dr. George Bonanno, a psychologist at Columbia University, has done research and written extensively on resilience to trauma. Although most of his work has been done with adults, his conclusions may be applicable to children as well. Bonanno notes first that resilience is different from recovery. Although resilient people may show transient responses to trauma, they maintain a stable equilibrium throughout and enjoy some protective factors that favor the development of positive outcomes and healthy personality characteristics.

Resilience is common and healthy and it comes in many forms. Bonanno calls these hardiness, self-enhancement, repressive coping, and positive emotion and laughter. While some of these are not generally viewed as positive attributes, they aid in adapting to trauma.

Hardy individuals are committed to finding a meaningful purpose in life, believe that one can influence his or her surroundings and the outcome of events, and believe that one can learn and grow from both positive and negative experiences. These people are not as threatened by traumatic situations, their distress is minimal, and they are more confident in seeking support.

While self-enhancement might be considered negative in some social contexts, a positive opinion of oneself, even to the point of narcissism, is helpful in the face of threat. Those who use repression as a coping mechanism routinely avoid unpleasant thoughts, emotions, and memories. This strategy may cause problems in some social situations but is adaptive in the context of trauma. Individuals who have a positive attitude, show gratitude and a genuine interest in the world, and love and frequently laugh fare better in dealing with stress. They believe that they can learn from it and grow.

These characteristics were found in adults. For children who have yet to develop a fixed personality style and coping mechanisms, a mix of factors including genetic predisposition, family interaction, and community support should be considered as well. There are many potential areas of research in understanding how all these factors are interrelated.

Psychiatrist David Charney at the National Institute of Mental Health has done extensive research in the psychobiological mechanisms of resilience and vulnerability. If people with post-traumatic stress disorder show an increase in brain norepinepherine and serotonin, decrease in hippocampal size, failed activation of the anterior cingulate cortex, and decreased serum cortisol levels, it might follow that resilient people show just the opposite findings. Animal and a few human studies have confirmed some of these hypotheses, but this is still a very new area of research.

The brain must be able to adapt to acute stress and then return to baseline function or homeostasis. If that base-line changes to a different set point, then the person will be more or less vulnerable to the next stressful episode. The resilient person quickly returns to or may not even leave the preexisting baseline level of response. Researchers have suggested many possible mechanisms to explain this. Perhaps there is a genetic difference in catecholamine or cortisol receptor density or receptor sensitivity. A person with fewer or less sensitive receptors would not be as vulnerable to the stress response. Conversely, more benzodiazepine receptors would facilitate calming.

Charney has suggested that the *allostatic load* may be important. The allostatic load is the cumulative physiologic burden borne by the body from attempts to adapt to stressors and the strains of life. Contributing to the load are eleven known neurochemical, neuropeptide, and hormonal mediators of the stress response (cortisol, dehydroandrosterone [DHEA], corticotropin-releasing hormone [CRH], locus coeruleus-norepinephrine system, neuropeptide Y, galanin, dopamine, serotonin, benzodiazepine receptors, testosterone, and estrogen). Individual levels or variable ratios and interactions may favor resilience or vulnerability.

A similar profile might be developed for psychological risk factors. These would include intelligence, effective self-regulation of emotions and attachment behaviors, positive self-concept, optimism, altruism, a capacity to convert traumatic helplessness into learned helpfulness, and an active coping style in confronting a stressor. To the extent that these traits can be learned or conditioned, that process would involve neural pathways. Brain-scanning techniques such as positron emission tomography (PET) can map function, and magnetic resonance imaging (MRI) the structures, of the brain. Neural circuits for reward, the conditioning and extinction of fear, and the formation of social attachments are most probably located in the amygdala. In resilient individuals, specific incoming stimuli are either not overgeneralized or are quickly extinguished. Reactivated memories are returned to long-term storage, a process that requires protein binding. Extinction—the repeated exposure to a stimulus without response—is facilitated, perhaps by more receptor sites. Cooperative social relationships are easier to forge. If specific neuronal pathways for these learning processes can be identified, specific genetic mechanisms in response to stress may be mapped and specific interventions developed. This work clearly confounds the notion of a mind-body dichotomy as more and more biological correlates of behavior are discovered.

## For Abusers

More genetic, hormonal, and structural work has been done with regard to susceptibility or resistance to stress disorders than to susceptibility or resistance to paraphilic disorders. Neuroimaging studies for differential arousal patterns would be of interest, as would hormonal and genetic studies.

It has been suggested that birth order may play a role in the development of pedophilia. This argument by analogy is based on the observation that, statistically, a subset of male homosexuals tends to have older brothers. The proposed mechanism is called maternal immunoreactivity. This would be similar to Rh and ABO blood group incompatibilities. In some pregnant women, the fetus provokes a maternal immune response so that maternal antibodies cross the placenta and affect the fetus. If the mother develops antibodies about some facet of maleness in the fetus, that response would increase with each subsequent male pregnancy. The maternal antibodies somehow disrupt neurohormonal development crucial for sexual differentiation of the fetal brain, and the male has female-type sexual preferences. If gender sexual preference can be disrupted in this way, why could age sexual preference not be disrupted in the same manner? Pedophiles should therefore, statistically, show a preponderance of men with older brothers. Some studies have shown this to be true. Disruptions leading to both homosexuality and pedophilia could independently occur in the same individual, but only in a small number of cases. Maternal immunoreactivity is likely to be just one of several factors contributing to sexual arousal to the young.

Several studies have reported an association, in men, between self-reported head injury before age thirteen and later pedophilic behavior. This could mean that subtle brain damage after birth increases the risk of pedophilia or that an as yet unknown neurodevelopmental problem before birth increases the risk of both accident-proneness and pedophilia. The correlation is not robust. Similarly, there are suggestions that pedophiles have a lower than expected level of intelligence, that they have a strong tendency to be left-handed, and that the first appearance of pedophilic behavior in an adult is associated with a temporal lobe disorder and/or an increased prolactin level. Large population studies with neuroimaging and sophisticated neuropsychological testing will be necessary to determine if these are, in fact, risk factors.

While developmental factors do seem to be more important than biological ones in the etiology of pedophilia, there may still be underlying neurophysiologic conditions that contribute to sexual arousal to children. Not every man exposed to the factors associated with such arousal becomes a pedophile. Some as yet unknown physiologic mechanism may make some individuals more susceptible or may even prevent the emergence of sexually abusive behavior in others.

Much work is yet to be done to understand both sides of the adult-child sexual experience. The ability to put aside prejudice and to be open to scientific inquiry is a prerequisite for any such work. Only in this way can we learn to be of help to those who are truly traumatized by the sexual experience rather than create additional "victims" with our own reactions and unhelpful interventions. We can work to identify and isolate those who will always present a danger to children—but also to identify and treat those who can be rehabilitated and become productive members of society.

# Appendix A

## State Sex Offender Registry Sites

These sites contain or have links to the relevant statutes and definitions.

Alabama
www.dps.state.al.us/public/abi/system/so

Alaska
www.dps.state.ak.us/nSorcr/asp

Arizona
www.az.gov/webapp/offender/main.do

Arkansas
www.acic.org/Registration/04-registered-sex-offenders.htm

California
www.caag.state.ca.us/megan

Colorado
www.sor.state.co.us/default.asp

Only serious offenders are online. Other requests go to local police departments.

Connecticut
www.state.ct.us/dps/Sex_Offender_Registry.htm

Delaware
www.state.de.us/dsp/sexoff/index.htm

District of Columbia
www.mpdc.dc.gov/serv/sor/sor.shtm

Florida
www3.fdle.state.fl.us/Sexual_Predators

Georgia
www.state.ga.us/gbi/disclaim.html

Hawaii
www.pahoehoe.ehawaii.gov/sexoff

Idaho
www.isp.state.id.us/identification/sex_offender/predator

Illinois
www.isp.state.il.us/sor/frames.htm

Indiana
www.state.in.us/serv/cji_sor

Iowa
www.iowasexoffender.com

Kansas
www.accesskansas.org/kbi/ro.shtml

Kentucky
kspsor.state.ky.us

Louisiana
www.lasocpr.lsp.org/socpr

Maine
www.informe.org/sor

Maryland
www.dpscs.state.md.us/onlineservs/sor

Massachusetts
www.mass.gov/sorb/community.htm

Michigan
www.mipsor.state.mi.us

Minnesota
www.doc.state.mn.us/level3/Search.asp

Mississippi
www.sor.mdps.state.ms.us

Missouri
www.mshp.dps.missouri.gov/MSHPWeb/PatrolDivision/
    CRID/SOR/SORPage.html

Montana
svor.doj.state.mt.us

Nebraska
www.nsp.state.ne.us/sor

Nevada
www.nvrepository.state.nv.us/Sexoffender.htm
Local police determine who may have access to this list.

New Hampshire
www.oit.nh.gov/nsor

New Jersey
www.njsp.org/info/reg_sexoffend.html

New Mexico
www.nmsexoffender.dps.state.nm.us

New York
criminaljustice.state.ny.us/nsor/index.htm

North Carolina
sbi.jus.state.nc.us/DOJHAHT/SOR/default.htm

North Dakota
www.ndsexoffender.com

Ohio
www.esorn.ag.state.oh.us/Secured/p1.aspx

Oklahoma
www.doc.state.ok.us/DOCS/offender_info.htm
Department of Corrections lists "habitual and aggravated" sex
  offenders.

Oregon
Oregon does not maintain an online registry. Call State Police
  for information.

Pennsylvania
www.psp.state.pa.us/psp/cwp/view.asp?a=3&q=150335

Puerto Rico
Puerto Rico does not maintain an online registry.

Rhode Island
Rhode Island does not maintain an online registry. RIS
  Chapter 11-37.1 describes the registration process.

South Carolina
www.sled.state.sc.us/SLED

South Dakota
dci.sd.gov/administration/id/sexoffender/index.asp

Tennessee
www.ticic.state.tn.us

Texas
records.txdps.state.tx.us/sosearch.cfm

Utah
www.udc.state.ut.us/asp-bin/sexoffendersearchform.asp

Vermont
www.dps.state.vt.us/cjs/s_registry.htm

Virginia
sex-offender.vsp.state.va.us/Static/cool-ICE

Washington
Washington does not maintain an online registry, but some
counties do. Release of information is at the discretion of
the local police.

West Virginia
www.wvstatepolice.com/sexoff

Wisconsin
offender.doc.state.wi.us/public/search/search.jsp

Wyoming
attorneygeneral.state.wy.us/dci/so/so_registration.html

# Appendix B

## Publications

Allgeier, E. R. & Allgeier, A. R. *Sexual Interactions*, 5th edition. Boston, Houghton Mifflin Co. 2000. A basic college textbook about human sexuality with a good section on sexual abuse.

American Psychiatric Association. *Diagnostic and Statistical Manual of Mental Disorders*, 4th edition. Washington, DC. 1994. Includes specific criteria for the diagnosis of each condition.

Bass, E. & Davis, L. *The Courage to Heal.* New York, Harper Collins. 1988. The book that started the repressed memory controversy.

Boyle, P. *Scouts Honor: Sexual Abuse in America's Most Trusted Institution.* Rocklin, CA, Prima Publishing. 1994. Sexual abuse in Scouting as told by participants.

Bremner, J. D. *Does Stress Damage the Brain? Understanding Trauma-Related Disorders from a Neurological Perspective.* New York, W. W. Norton & Co. 2002. Focus on damage to the hippocampus.

Carr, C. *The Alienist.* New York, Random House. 1994. A fictionalized account of child prostitution in New York City in 1896.

Courtois, C. *Recollections of Sexual Abuse: Treatment Principles and Guidelines.* New York, W. W. Norton & Co. 1999. Evolving standards of practice in working with those who may have been abused.

Follette, V. M., Ruzek, J. J. & Abueg, F. R. (eds.). *Cognitive-Behavioral Therapies for Trauma.* New York, Guilford. 1998. Description of various techniques by experts in each.

Friedman, M. J., Charney, D. S. & Deutch, A. Y. (eds.). *Neurological and Clinical Consequences of Stress: From Normal Adaptation to Post-Traumatic Stress Disorder.* Philadelphia, Lippincott. 1995. A collection of relevant studies.

Herman, J. *Trauma and Recovery.* New York, Basic Books. 1992. The classic description of the recovery process.

Laumann, E. O., Gagnon, J. H., Michael, R. T. & Michaels, S. *The Social Organization of Sexuality: Sexual Practices in the United States.* Chicago, University of Chicago Press. 1994. The most extensive field study done in the United States.

Loftus, E. & Ketcham, K. *The Myth of Repressed Memory: False Memories and Allegations of Sexual Abuse.* New York, St. Martin's Griffin. 1996. An expert in memory looks at the controversy.

Resick, P. A. *Stress and Trauma.* Philadelphia, Taylor and Francis. 2001. An excellent treatment resource.

Shapiro, F. *Eye Movement Desensitization and Reprocessing: Basic Principles, Protocols, and Procedures.* New York, Guilford. 1995. A description of this therapeutic approach by its founder.

Sipe, A. W. R. *Celibacy in Crisis.* New York, Brunner-Routledge. 2003. A look at the sexual behavior of Catholic priests.

Van der Kolk, B. A., McFarlane, A. C. & Weisarth, L. (eds.). *Traumatic Stress: The Effects of Overwhelming Experience on Mind, Body, and Society.* New York, Guilford. 1996. Includes several relevant chapters.

# Appendix C

## The Internet

Stop It Now!
www.stopitnow.com
Sponsors a helpline for abusers, 888-PREVENT

Sex Addicts Anonymous
www.sexaa.org
Twelve-step program with over 500 meetings around the
world, 800-477-8191

Sexuality Education and Information Council of the United
States (SIECUS)
www.siecus.org
Fact sheets and annotated bibliographies about sexual abuse.

American Association of Sex Educators, Counselors, and
Therapists (AASECT)
www.aasect.org
Includes listing of certified sex therapists.

National Center for the Prosecution of Child Abuse
www.ndaa-apri.org/apri/programs/ncpca/ncpca_home.html
Trains prosecutors with reference to all relevant state statues.

VIRTUS
www.virtusonline.org
Produces and updates the Protecting God's Children program
for the Catholic Church.

PubMed
www.ncbi.nlm.nih.gov
National Library of Medicine search service with over eleven
million resources.

Open-Mind
www.open-mind.org
Includes an online Survivors Forum.

Survivors Network of Those Abused by Priests
www.snapnetwork.org
For self-help, education, and prevention with fifty support
groups nationwide.

New Hampshire Coalition Against Domestic and Sexual
Violence
www.nhcadsv.org
A representative state group stressing service to victims, education, and accountability.

California Attorney General www.caag.state.ca.us/
childabuse
Guidelines for protection as well as legal remedies.

Computer Retrieval of Information on Scientific Projects
www.crisp.cit.nih.gov
Information about all grant projects currently funded by the
National Institutes of Health. Search for "child sexual abuse."

MedLinePlus
www.medlineplus.gov
Online medical encyclopedia and dictionary.

# Glossary

**Addiction**   Psychological or physiological dependence on a substance or practice that is beyond voluntary control.

**Adrenal glands**   A pair of small glands that sit upon the kidneys and produce cortisol in the outer layer (adrenal cortex) and adrenalin in the central area (adrenal medulla).

**Adrenalin (Epinephrine)**   A catecholamine secreted by the adrenal medulla and by neurons in the central nervous system. It increases the rate and strength of the heartbeat and dilates small arteries within muscle tissue.

**Amygdala**   A cluster of specialized nerve cells deep in each hemisphere that plays an important role in emotions.

**Autonomic nervous system**   That part of the nervous system that innervates smooth muscle, cardiac muscle, and gland cells. It has two divisions: the sympathetic increases activity and the parasympathetic promotes rest and restoration.

**Aversive conditioning**   Techniques that pair a painful, noxious, or otherwise unwelcome stimulus with particular thoughts or behaviors in order to extinguish them.

**Biofeedback**   Technique where changes in unconscious or involuntary body functions are made perceptible to the senses in order to modulate them by conscious mental control.

**Brain stem**   Portion of the central nervous system that connects spinal cord with brain and contains many nerve cells that regulate primitive brain function.

**Castration**   Removal of the testicles or ovaries.

**Catecholamine**   A class of neurotransmitters that includes epinephrine, norepinephrine, and L-dopa.

**Celibacy**   Complete sexual abstinence.

**Cerebellum**   Part of the brain that coordinates muscle tone, posture, and eye and hand movements based on sensory information received from other parts of the brain.

**Cerebral cortex**   Outer layer and major portion of the brain; contains nerve cells for speech, motor activity, sensory reception, emotion, and cognitive functions.

**Cognition**   The mental activities associated with thinking, learning, and memory.

**Cognitive behavioral therapy**   Form of therapy that combines verbal communication and behavioral techniques in order to affect change.

**Comorbidity**   The coexistence of two or more unrelated disease processes.

**Cortisol**   Hormone produced by the adrenal cortex that affects the metabolism of glucose, protein, and fat; often increases in response to stress.

**Countertransference**   Therapist's responses to a client based on the therapist's past experiences or response to the patient's transference.

**Covert sensitization**   A behavioral technique using imagination alone to affect change.

**Debriefing**   Talking about a traumatic experience immediately after it occurs.

**Depersonalization**   A state in which one loses the feeling of one's own identity.

**Desensitization**   The reduction or elimination of reactions to a specific stimulus.

**Deviation**   A departure from an accepted norm, role, or rule.

**Dissociation**   An unconscious separation of one group of mental processes from the others.

**Dyspareunia**   The occurrence of pain on the part of the woman during sexual intercourse.

**Dysphoria**   A feeling of unpleasantness or discomfort.

**EMDR (Eye movement desensitization and reprocessing)**   A therapeutic technique where rapid eye movement is paired with repeated traumatic images and positive affirmations.

**Enabler**   A person who tacitly supports or ignores negative behavior in another, thereby allowing or encouraging it to continue.

**Endocrine glands**   The glands in the body that secrete hormones which affect the function of other parts of the body.

**Ephebophilia**   A paraphilia in which there is sexual attraction to postpubescent youths.

**Extinction**   The progressive decrease in the frequency of a response that is no longer positively reinforced.

**Fixation**   A firm attachment to a particular person or object from an earlier period of one's development.

**Flooding**   A behavioral technique in which clients immerse themselves in their most anxiety-producing situations.

**Galvanic skin response (GSR)**   The measurement of variation in skin conductance due to sympathetically driven increase in perspiration.

**Global Positioning System (GPS)**   A system that pinpoints geographic location via satellite tracking.

**Hippocampus**   The seahorse-shaped structure in the cerebral cortex that is part of the limbic system; connects with brain stem nuclei as well.

**Hormone**   A chemical substance formed in one organ of the body and carried in the blood to alter the function of another organ.

**Hypnosis**   An induced trancelike state during which the subject is highly suggestible.

**Hypothalamus**   Part of the brain stem composed of multiple nerve centers; coordinates and controls body functions such as eating, sleeping, and sexual behavior, maintains body temperature and chemical balance, and regulates many hormones.

**Incest**   Sexual relations between persons closely related by blood.

**Limbic system**   An interrelated circuit of deep brain structures involved in emotion, behavior, autonomic function, and smell.

**Locus coeruleus**   A cell cluster in the wall of the fourth ventricle of the brain whose norepinephrine-containing axons have wide distribution in the cerebellum, hypothalamus, and cerebral cortex.

**Magnetic resonance imaging (MRI)**   A method of body scanning that can be used to detect abnormalities of structure within the brain.

**Masturbation**   The self-stimulation of the genitals for erotic pleasure and orgasm.

**Meta-analysis**   The process of using statistical methods to combine the results of different studies.

**Neurobiology**   The biology of the nervous system.

**Neuroimaging**   Techniques used to visualize the function or anatomy of the central nervous system.

**Neurotransmitter**   A chemical that functions within the nervous system as part of the process of transmitting information from one neuron to the next.

**Noradrenalin (norepinephrine)**   A catecholamine that serves as the primary neurotransmitter within the sympathetic nervous system.

**Pap test**   A cervical smear examined for abnormal cells, named for Dr. George Papanicolaou.

**Paraphilia**   A condition of compulsive responsivity to and obligatory dependence on an unusual and socially unacceptable external stimulus or internal fantasy for sexual arousal.

**Pedophilia**   A paraphilia in which there is sexual attraction to prepubescent youths.

**Penile plethysmograph**   A device to measure changes in the volume of the penis.

**Pituitary**   A gland on the underside of the brain that produces neurohormones which assist in the regulation of hormone production by other glands.

**Plea-bargain**   A legal maneuver where the designated offense and punishment are agreed upon by the prosecution and defense in order to avoid or end a trial.

**Polygraph**   An instrument to measure changes in respiration, blood pressure, and galvanic skin response (GSR) while the subject is being questioned about emotionally charged topics.

**Pornography**   Sexually explicit material designed for arousal.

**Positron emission tomography (PET)**   A method of body scanning using mildly radioactive compounds to yield images of activity level.

**Post-traumatic stress disorder (PTSD)**   The reexperience of trauma, avoidance of associated stimuli, and increased agitation following a traumatic incident.

**Prostate-specific antigen (PSA)**   A substance that induces a state of sensitivity; elevated in diseases of the prostate.

**Psychopathology**   A general term for mental and behavioral disorders.

**Psychotherapy**   The treatment of mental distress through verbal communication.

**Puberty**   The phase of life, usually in adolescence, where reproductive fertility and physical changes consistent with sexual maturity begin.

**Rapid eye movement (REM)**   The stage of sleep where the eyes move rapidly beneath closed lids, the body does not move, and dreaming occurs.

**Recidivism**   A relapse to a previous behavior pattern.

**Regression**   The return to a more primitive mode of behavior.

**Repression**   The active process of keeping memories out of conscious awareness.

**Resilience**   The ability to recover from or adjust easily to a traumatic experience.

**Separation anxiety**   A developmental stage (usually between eight and fourteen months of age) during which a child experiences anxiety when separated from the primary caregiver (usually the mother).

**Serotonin**   A monoamine that serves as a neurotransmitter in the central nervous system.

**Somatization**   The process by which psychological needs are expressed as physical symptoms.

**Testosterone**   The most potent androgenic hormone, formed mostly in the testes.

**Therapeutic community**   A milieu where patients and staff together make important decisions about community life.

**Transference**   The projection of feelings, thoughts, and wishes onto the therapist as representative of a person from the patient's past.

**Vaginismus**   Painful spasm of the vagina.

**Ventricle**   One of a system of communicating cavities within the brain.

# Index

Understanding Health and Sickness Series
*Miriam Bloom, Ph.D., General Editor*

**Also in this series**